IT WORKS FOR ME!

IT WORKS FOR ME!

CELEBRITY STORIES OF ALTERNATIVE HEALING

HEIDE BANKS

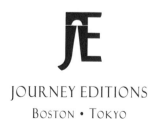

JOURNEY EDITIONS

BOSTON • TOKYO

First published in 1996 by Journey Editions,
an imprint of Charles E. Tuttle Co., Inc. of Rutland, Vermont and Tokyo, Japan,
with editorial offices at 153 Milk Street, Boston, Massachusetts 02109

© 1996 Heide Banks
Published by Ottenheimer Publishers, Inc.
10 Church Lane, Baltimore, Maryland 21208
ME-004A

CIP data for this book is available from the Library of Congress.

ISBN 1-885203-31-4
1 3 5 7 9 10 8 6 4 2

Printed in the United States of America

*For Laird Cagan and Jan Shepherd
without whose support, encouragement, and faith
this book would never have been possible.*

And to all those who have made healing a priority in their lives.

NOTE TO THE READER

The information in *It Works for Me!* is designed to help increase your knowledge of alternative healing techniques that may relieve health problems in some cases. This book is intended as a reference resource only, and does not purport to give medical advice. Do not use any alternative healing technique in this book without first consulting your physician or in place of prompt and proper medical care. The information contained in this book is not intended to substitute for the advice of your physician or any treatment that he or she may prescribe or recommend. Instead, use this book as a complement to your cooperative relationship with your physician.

CONTENTS

FOREWORD

Writing *Chicken Soup for the Soul* and *A 2nd Helping of Chicken Soup for the Soul* has changed my life in many ways. For the past twenty years my life as an educator and lecturer has kept me very busy traveling and teaching, but with the success of these books I found myself on the road more than ever, traveling from city to city, usually without my family and on less sleep than I would have liked.

However, all the time I spent on the road was more than compensated for by the people I met and the stories they shared with me about how they had overcome the obstacles and hardships in their lives by transforming them into building blocks. I came to appreciate just how powerful a role inspirational stories, not unlike those contained in *It Works For Me!*, can play in empowering people to create more productive, healthy, and rewarding lives.

No matter how many stories I heard, I was always deeply touched by how each of these people had found the courage to face challenges and turn their lives around. What they all seemed to possess was a gratitude for being alive and for being able to make a contribution to others. They had all made a decision to do the very best they could with what they had available to them at the time.

A perfect example of this is the story of W. Mitchell, who as a result of a terrible motorcycle accident was burned beyond recognition on over 65 percent of his body. Sixteen surgeries later, Mitchell was left unable to dial a phone, get himself to the bathroom, or pick up a fork. But, six months after that, he was piloting a plane.

Four years after his accident, Mitchell's plane crashed, leaving him permanently paralyzed from the waist down. Still, Mitchell went on to serve as mayor of his town, run for Congress, fall in love, get married, earn a master's degree, and become a millionaire.

His unshakably positive mental attitude and his gratitude for what he has accomplished have fueled Mitchell's life. Mitchell readily admits there were 10,000 things he could do before his accidents and now there are only 9,000. But, instead of dwelling on the 1,000 he can't do, he chooses to focus on the 9,000 that are left. As Mitchell likes to say, "It's not what happens to you in life, it's what you choose to do about it that makes the difference."

Clearly Mitchell's story is a dramatic one, but what it illustrates is that no matter what happens to you physically, you can always fight back and create a life that is fulfilling and productive. Mitchell's accidents left him with lifelong conditions to which he had to adjust; however, many people who contract even serious illnesses can actually recreate total health. This has even been documented with HIV-positive individuals who have used alternative therapies and holistic approaches to help stave off the onset of AIDS indefinitely.

While you read the stories that follow in *It Works For Me!* and learn of the challenges each of these celebrated people faced, and the triumphs they created, remember that whatever methods you choose to enhance your health and overall well-being, it's equally important to reach out with gratitude and love for the life you have been blessed with and for those who are around you. This is perhaps the greatest medicine of them all.

Jack Canfield
Co-Author, *Chicken Soup for the Soul*

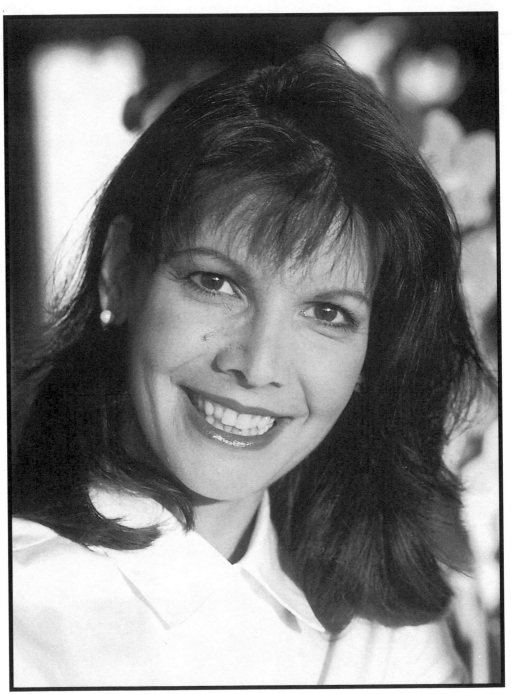

Pablo Anleu

INTRODUCTION

The day my phone rang and the voice on the other end asked if I wanted to write a book on alternative healing, a subject I passionately believed in, I was convinced it was God disguising his voice to sound like a Baltimore-based publisher.

I knew I'd enjoy writing this book. What I never expected was the healing I would receive as a result. Given my health record, this was no easy feat. While I'd done the best with the body I was given, something always seemed to be tugging away at my health.

The stress I put myself under never helped the situation much. Something about every project I took on—from producing television shows to home decorating—left me exhausted and sick. But this project was turning out differently. With every day I spent on it, I felt healthier.

Don't get me wrong. This was not a simple project. Finding eighteen celebrated people willing to candidly discuss some very vulnerable areas in their lives proved to be quite a challenge.

But I found that by using the information I was gathering for this book to work through my challenges, I was able to experience healing in a new and deeper way. As a result, the year I spent writing became the healthiest year of my life.

It had a lot to do with the inspiration I received from the celebrities I was writing about. The strength and courage it took for them to deal with their own challenges moved me to find my own. When actor Dirk Benedict told me what it was like to wake up filled with cancer, feeling that anything less than a 100 percent commitment to his healing process could result in death, I was inspired to make an even deeper commitment to my own healing process.

I felt gratitude for my health the day sweetly shy animator Phyllis Bird visited my mountaintop home. Inspired by the view, Birdie, as I had come to know her, shared with me what it felt like to be told she'd have to give up her lifelong passion—painting the mystical scenery and creatures in Disney movies—because of the infection that was ravishing her artists' hands.

It made it easier knowing others were facing similar challenges in their lives. When Mike Farrell spoke to me of his family's legacy of poor health, I was reminded of my own. As a family, we were gifted with many wonderful assets—courage, humor, and abundantly thick hair—but what we all seemed to lack was robust health.

Many members of my family died prematurely. I was lucky to briefly know two of my grandparents: Ruth, my father's mother, who lived out her years shuffling between hospitals and nursing homes; and Grandpa Joe, my mother's father.

Grandpa Joe led an active life as an entertainer on the road with his brother. Those two were inseparable. And, apart from his dependency on an over-the-counter stomach remedy, Grandpa Joe was in fine health. Then, his brother died. Their act was over, and Joe's health took a serious nosedive. Just four months to the day after his brother passed on, Joe followed him.

This left an impression on me. For once, everyone in my feisty family was in agreement—what killed Grandpa Joe wasn't bad health but a broken heart. It was my first experience of the powerful connection between mind, body and spirit—the underlying principle of alternative health care.

But it still would be many years before I would come to fully understand just how powerful a connection this can be.

Like others I interviewed for this book, such as award-winning novelist Alice Walker, whose natural curiosity led her to try Watsu, an alternative therapy that asks you to place your vulnerability into the hands of a stranger, my own spirit of adventure led me to alternative healing.

My formal introduction came through a chiropractor who used a few simple exercises along with a spinal adjustment to help correct my perplexing, lifelong inability to distinguish between my left and right sides. Before his help I hadn't been able to tell without raising my hand to recite the pledge of allegiance!

While I appreciated this new sense of direction, I had to admit it wasn't life-changing enough to get me to abandon conventional health care.

By this time, I was living in Los Angeles, a mecca for alternative practitioners and all the latest healing techniques. I continued to experiment with many of the alternative methods you'll read about in this book. I was Rolfed and acupunctured. I took up meditation, attended personal growth seminars, and finally made the ultimate sacrifice. I traded in my aluminum cookware, which many alternative health practitioners decry as a source of poisoning, for nontoxic, alternatively correct pots and pans.

But I wasn't about to give up my frenetic pace. I continued to stress out over work, relationships and life in general. Each time, I turned to alternative medicine to restore my health. However, I treated it no differently than I had conventional medicine—I expected instant, spontaneous relief. Whenever some alternative therapy demanded a change in my lifestyle or a greater commitment than swallowing a remedy, I'd fall back on conventional approaches. The familiar route just seemed easier. All that changed when I found myself in the hospital, hooked up to IVs—intravenous lines.

Like long-distance swimmer Diana Nyad's emergency throat surgery and actress Sally Kirkland's near-death experience, it took a life-threatening situation for me to fully embrace alternative healing.

I had contracted pleurisy, a kind of pneumonia that fills the membrane around the lungs with excess fluid. In the hospital, I was given intravenous medications for the infection and morphine for the pain. But how, I kept asking the physicians, *how did this happen to me?* I thought I had been taking good care of myself, eating well, exercising, getting lots of rest. Their answer? Never mind how—the solution was surgery and two months on IVs.

This was my wake-up call. Finally, I was ready to admit that I could no longer ignore the mind, body, and spirit connection. I knew then it wasn't the stress in my life that was affecting me, but the way I was reacting to the stress. I believed then, and do now, that it was slowly killing me.

I began to make the changes my alternative practitioners had been suggesting all along. Mostly, I began to treat myself better. I stopped making everything—relationships, career, deadlines—more important than loving and nurturing myself. And I soon discovered what medical studies have already confirmed. People who feel loved and supported, people who remain calmer during periods of emotional upset, and people who are optimistic can achieve greater health.

I became more realistic about what my body could endure, admitting that while I was stronger than ever, that was no excuse to try to push my body past its limits. And when at times I did become sick, instead of judging myself, I deliberately adopted an attitude of compassion. Essentially, I "loved myself healthy." This represented a major change for me.

My story's not unique. As you read about the challenges each of these celebrities faced and how they used alternative healing to create better lives, you'll notice a number of similarities.

They were all willing to try something new—recognizing first that what they had been doing could be improved upon. And as they explored each alternative therapy, they were careful to use everything they learned. They recognized that in whatever area the challenge lay—health, relationships, career or finances—there was an opportunity both to cure the problem and at the same time to enhance the quality of their lives. This attitude resulted in profound and lasting results.

Often, it was as important to give up what wasn't working for them as it was to try something new. This was the case with Morgan Fairchild, whose bout with chronic fatigue taught her that sometimes the greatest therapy is just learning to say no to things that are too stressful. While they looked to alternative healing for answers, they also learned to embrace the challenges they faced, creating healing in the process.

Kenny Loggins was one of the final interviews I conducted for this book. When I arrived at his beachfront home I realized that I was physically and emotionally exhausted. Mounting deadlines and holiday pressures were having their way with me, and I needed rest and nurturing to get back into balance.

But as I sat there talking with Kenny and his wife, Julia, something began to shift. I found myself relaxing into the warmth and support that surrounded this loving family and almost magically, I felt my body start to heal and come back into alignment. When I left there hours later, I knew I was healthier than when I had arrived.

How perfect that this was to be my final interview. After exploring everything from acupuncture to yoga, I realized there was one method of alternative healing I hadn't touched on: *surrounding yourself with love.*

As you read through this book, I make but one suggestion: to use this most powerful method of healing as often and as completely as possible.

Heide Banks
Santa Barbara, California

ABOUT THE AUTHOR

Heide Banks is an author, lecturer, and frequent guest on both radio and television. She has appeared on such shows as *Good Day New York, ABC News,* and *The Leeza Show.*

An avid student of alternative methods of healing and well-being, Heide served as a board member for The Center for Health, a major alternative healing center in Los Angeles. Her extensive lecturing and work on the healing power of interpersonal relationships has led her to be dubbed "The Deepak of Dating." She currently lectures and conducts workshops throughout the country.

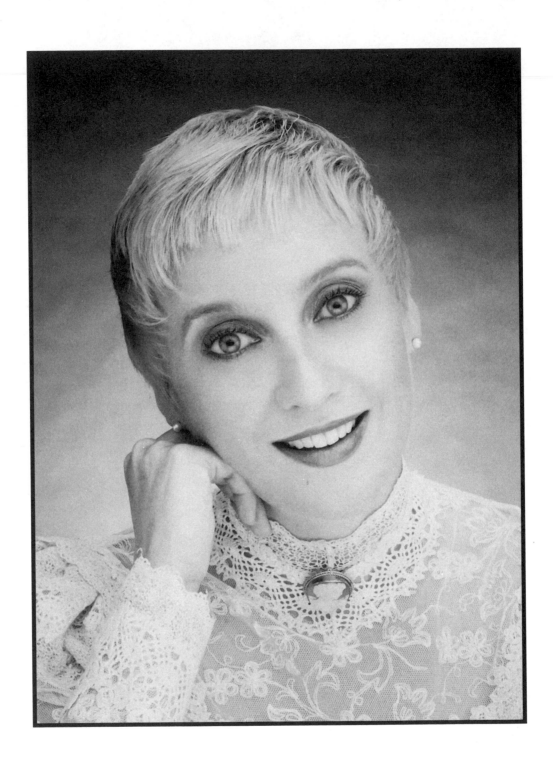

1 ACUPUNCTURE

BORN
June 22, 1953,
Granite City, Illinois

EDUCATION
B.A., College of Wooster
M.S., University of Illinois
at Champagne

PROFESSIONAL AWARDS
Grammy, 1987: *Bernstein's Candide*,
New World Records

CAREER HIGHLIGHTS
PERFORMANCES
Houston Opera—debut
Metropolitan Opera
La Scala
Chicago Lyric Opera
New York City Opera
Santa Fe Opera
L'Opera de Montreal
Chamber Music Society at
Lincoln Center

RECORDINGS
Muzio
Follies
Candide

"I get my body into such good shape with acupuncture that bad stuff can't come in."

At barely a tiara past five feet tall, forty-two-year-old opera star Erie Mills is known around the world for her soaring coloratura and sparkling energy. She spends more than 200 days a year on the road, playing such roles as the flirtatious Rosina in *Barber of Seville,* the humorous Marie in *Daughter of the Regiment,* and the exhibitionist Olympia in *Tales of Hoffmann*; music critics from New York to Santa Fe call her a "brilliant singer, thoughtful musician, [and] convincing actor."

But don't look to Erie for the larger-than-life diva attitude that frequently comes with those kinds of reviews. Even though a singer's life on the road can be grueling, she never complains. Erie gives everything *but* attitude to each performance, no matter how she feels.

Yet the 1990–91 opera season, between September and June, was a particularly taxing one, even for a trooper like Erie. "I was sick with a sore throat an average of once a month," says Erie. "I flushed a lot of liquids down to try and get rid of the infection that caused it, but the infection went into my sinuses. Then my sinuses

1

started to drain, and I began to cough and have chest pains. So it was not only in my throat but also in my head and chest.

"I realize that there are gradations of not feeling well," adds Erie. "But while for others a little bit of a cold may not be much, for opera singers it can be a disaster."

Despite all she was suffering, Erie kept up her travel schedule. "I would fly into a city and see a doctor who would prescribe antibiotics. The drugs would work for a while, but then I would go on to the next job, where I would get sick again."

Clearly, bouncing around from city to city, doctor to doctor, and antibiotic to antibiotic was not the best way to get well. Or to live.

Yet this is where Erie found herself at the end of the 1990–91 opera season. She had just realized every opera singer's dream and debuted at the Metropolitan Opera House in New York, then rushed off to a singing engagement in Santa Fe. And, once again, she was ill. "I don't remember much about the trip except that I was on antibiotics and not feeling my best," Erie recalls. "I was en route to Santa Fe with a number of stopovers. Many singers won't fly when they're ill. Their doctors tell them not to. To singers, flying is always miserable because of the dry air and pressure on your ears."

But Erie was expected in Santa Fe to star in a production as part of the summer opera season. She was to sing the title role in *Die Schweigsame en Frau*, a complex operatic piece that critics say places unusually heavy demands upon even the most accomplished of singers.

Ironically, the English translation of this Strauss opera is *The Silent Woman*, a real-life role Erie might have been forced to play had her various problems persisted.

"This was a big role, even for me," Erie says. "Even though it was called *The Silent Woman*, the woman I play is not very silent. She sings all night long."

Fortunately, there was a rehearsal period, which gave Erie an opportunity to get in better shape before opening night.

"When I first arrived in Santa Fe for rehearsal, I was coughing and blowing my nose all the time," Erie says. "I was mentally drained and so tired of being sick."

Obviously sympathetic to her suffering, two fellow cast members approached Erie and suggested she see an acupuncturist they knew in Santa Fe. "At this point, I was so sick that I was willing to try anything," Erie says.

Erie knew little about acupuncture, the Chinese alternative therapy that uses sterilized, disposable needles as thin as a hair to redirect what they call *qi* or *chi*, life energy, along fourteen pathways called meridians that, according to traditional Chinese medicine, exist throughout the body. Inserted into any number of 400 different points along these paths, the needles are thought to balance the flow of energy and restore health.

"When I first went to see the acupuncturist I was feeling lousy," says the singer. "I was still ill, and my antibiotics had run out." But Erie went to his office in a little house in downtown Santa Fe. The front of the house is a mini health food store where he sells herbal remedies, and the back contains rooms for acupuncture.

Not knowing what to expect, Erie ventured in. At first she and the acupuncturist just talked. "He was very considerate," recalls Erie. "First he told me a little about what to expect, then I told him my medical history and what had been going on."

After their conversation, Erie got up on a padded table in the middle of the room. The acupuncturist diagnosed her condition by taking her pulse twice, then told her that weak organs were causing the chronic infections that had been plaguing her.

The next thing Erie knew, the acupuncturist was sticking needles all over her tiny body. "He put about ten or twelve needles at different points on my body," says the singer. "He put most of the needles in my hands, ankles, and elbows. It didn't hurt at all. I felt very relaxed and I slept through half of the treatment."

Before Erie left the acupuncturist's house, he also prescribed some herbs. Although Erie didn't know what herbs they were, the acupuncturist assured her that supplementing acupuncture with herbs would bolster the effects of her treatment.

THE SILENT WOMAN SINGS

That afternoon was the first rehearsal day for Erie and the opera company. Even though she wouldn't be expected to sing, Erie *would* be expected to remain onstage for the entire rehearsal period—well over four hours.

Erie arrived at the opera house not knowing how her sick body was going to do it. "It was a blocking rehearsal, where the director tells each of us where to sit or stand at different points throughout the opera." At one point, "I was staged to be sitting and sewing," says Erie. "The director went off to talk to someone else in the cast, and I found myself drifting off. I was so relaxed that I fell off my chair. I went straight over before I caught myself. I thought, 'Oh my goodness, I'm really tired.'"

Erie told the acupuncturist what had happened. "He told me that this was a common reaction to acupuncture treatments—that you get tired, especially if your body is releasing a lot of bad stuff."

But aside from her tiredness, Erie was on the road to recovery. "I started feeling better" almost immediately, says Erie. "Singing is about the physical being. Singers don't have an instrument like a violinist. We don't pick a violin out of a case and start playing it. Our instrument is on the inside, our voice. So if you are not feeling well, your voice will not be in the best of shape. But if you are feeling well, then you can do what you are trained to do."

That's exactly what Erie did opening night. She had the audience at her feet, and critics applauded her "awesome singing talent" and "fierce energy."

Fortunately for Erie, she was to remain in Santa Fe for the remainder of the summer—the next eight weeks. "The first couple of weeks, I saw the acupuncturist about three times a week," says the singer. While focusing upon acupuncture treatments, he also suggested various herbs to help strengthen her organs further. Soon, Erie was able to reduce her acupuncture to a weekly "maintenance" visit.

By the end of the summer when Erie was ready to leave Santa Fe, there was no longer the remotest need for antibiotics.

RETURN TO SANTA FE

Erie's Santa Fe performances were so successful that she found herself invited back to Santa Fe two summers later. "Santa Fe hired me for the summers of 1993 and 1994," says the singer. "When I got there in 1993, I was feeling good. I had been exercising a lot more, I had continued with my herbs, and I had not been sick."

Once back in town, Erie signed up for a series of acupuncture maintenance treatments—just for insurance. "I had one treatment per week the whole ten weeks I was there," she says. "I went to each treatment feeling pretty healthy, but I think there were probably some weaknesses caused by flying and stress that the acupuncturist worked on.

"Each session was very similar. The acupuncturist began by taking my pulse and ended by sticking needles in different parts of my body. Again, I found it very relaxing and managed to fall asleep during the treatments.

"I remember one session in which he said to me, 'Your kidneys seem to be a little inflamed today.' Actually, I had been out the night before drinking margaritas with Mexican food. I found it amazing that he could see that in me so quickly."

Erie, now a regular at the Santa Fe festival each summer, scheduled follow-up treatments the next summer as well. "I think of it as storing up good things," Erie says. "I get my body in such good shape through acupuncture that bad stuff can't come in. I use it in a preventive way."

But after a summer season of feeling great, last fall Erie arrived in Montreal and got sick. "I panicked," says the singer. "I wanted to nip it in the bud so that all of my performances could go on as scheduled. So I went back to a physician and took my first antibiotic since 1991.

"I probably would have been fine not taking them," Erie says. "But sometimes we just don't trust our bodies to allow them to heal themselves.

"But acupuncture has taught me that there are alternatives that work," adds the singer. "I think the year I spent on antibiotics really depleted my body and worked against my immune system. It took some time for me to realize it, but the truth is that the body is an incredible thing, and if we allow it to take care of itself, it usually will."

Getting ready to board a plane bound for a singing engagement in Japan, Erie says that lesson will keep her happy and in good health on the coming tour. Nevertheless, along with her two personal physicists—her husband, physicist Thomas Rescigno, and Fermi, their Toto-like cairn terrier, who is named for the physicist Enrique Fermi—Erie has a brand-new copy of *Fodor's Guidebook*. It will help her scout out restaurants, shrines, and temples—and a good acupuncturist, should the need arise.

SPOTLIGHT ON ACUPUNCTURE

It's hard to argue about a medical treatment that's been around for over 5,000 years and boasts billions of satisfied consumers. So while the day is still pretty far off when you'll be calling your doctor to complain of a nagging headache only to be told to take two needles and call back in the morning, it shouldn't be too surprising that the 9,000 acupuncturists in the United States reported that they scheduled over ten million patient visits in 1993 alone.

Acupuncture is clearly poking its way into mainstream medical care. But you've got to wonder just what makes people want to have hair-thin needles stuck under their skin.

It apparently began in the mid-1800s, when acupuncture was brought to America by Chinese immigrants, but it did not become popular until 1972, when columnist James Reston of the *New York Times* was forced to undergo an emergency appendectomy while traveling in China. The appendectomy went well and Reston was treated to a few well-placed acupuncture needles afterward to relieve his pain. He wrote about the experience, igniting America's curiosity about acupuncture.

As China began to open its doors to Americans over the next few years, American doctors were able to visit Chinese hospitals and see acupuncture practiced firsthand. The Americans found that the Chinese doctors had developed a complex body map that conceptualized the human body as a system of twelve major pathways, called meridians. Each meridian is linked to a specific organ within the body, and each has nearly a hundred acupuncture points along its length. According to Chinese teachings, when acupuncture needles are inserted into these points, they are able to eliminate any blockages on the meridian by redirecting and increasing the flow of *qi* or *chi*—the Chinese word for "energy" or "life force." When someone's *chi* is blocked or out of balance, pain and disease are the result.

Some researchers theorize that when a needle is inserted into a particular point in the body, it stimulates the release of endorphins, the body's natural painkillers. Others feel that when a needle is inserted, it overloads the body's pain circuits and simply shuts them down.

However it works, acupuncture has been used for centuries to counteract everything from arthritis and asthma to chronic pain and PMS. More recently it has found another audience in treating addictions, from cigarettes to heroin.

If you decide to consult an acupuncturist, expect your initial consultation to begin with the acupuncturist giving your body a once-over. The acupuncturist will look at your tongue for any coating and your skin to study your coloring. At the same time, he'll ask you questions about diet, exercise, any sensitivities to heat or cold and, of course, your medical history.

All the while he'll listen to the strength and tone of your voice—all signals these physicians are trained to interpret when diagnosing a patient. Finally the doctor will feel your pulse, determining the strength of the signal. But if you are expecting him or her to stop at one wrist, you may be surprised. Acupuncturists believe that every person actually has twelve pulse points, and checking at least two of them is critical to reaching an accurate diagnosis.

Once satisfied with the diagnosis, the acupuncturist will then ask you to lie down on the table while he begins to insert needles at critical points throughout your body. The needles are thin, sterilized stainless steel shafts that can be disposed of after your treatment. You might find a few on your hands, or just above your temples or above the bridge of your nose. It all depends on what organ the acupuncturist is trying to reach.

How long the needle remains in is based on the problem, or "imbalance," the acupuncturist has found. It can last anywhere from a few seconds to an hour, but generally expect a session to last half an hour. And don't worry about the pain. You may feel an initial pricking and perhaps an ache, but that should be all. If you feel any more than that, alert the acupuncturist. He or she will simply change the needle's direction, and any discomfort should immediately be alleviated.

Depending on the nature and severity of your problem, it may take one or more acupuncture sessions to solve it. Many acupuncturists will ask you to return three or four times the first week, cutting back to one visit a week thereafter. After the problem is solved, a maintenance program of once a month may be suggested, or a seasonal "tune-up" may be recommended to assure continued good health.

If a medical problem is such that it can only be corrected by surgery, then acupuncture may be used to speed recovery and help with any pain or discomfort you may be feeling.

However you choose to use acupuncture, make sure you check the credentials of your acupuncturist first.

For acupuncturists who are not medical doctors, twenty-five states set rigorous training standards and then license those who meet them. These states are Alaska, California, Colorado, Florida, Hawaii, Iowa, Louisiana, Maine, Maryland, Massachusetts, Montana, Nevada, New Jersey, New Mexico, New York, North Carolina, Oregon, Pennsylvania, Rhode Island, Texas, Utah, Vermont, Virginia, Washington, and Wisconsin, as well as the District of Columbia.

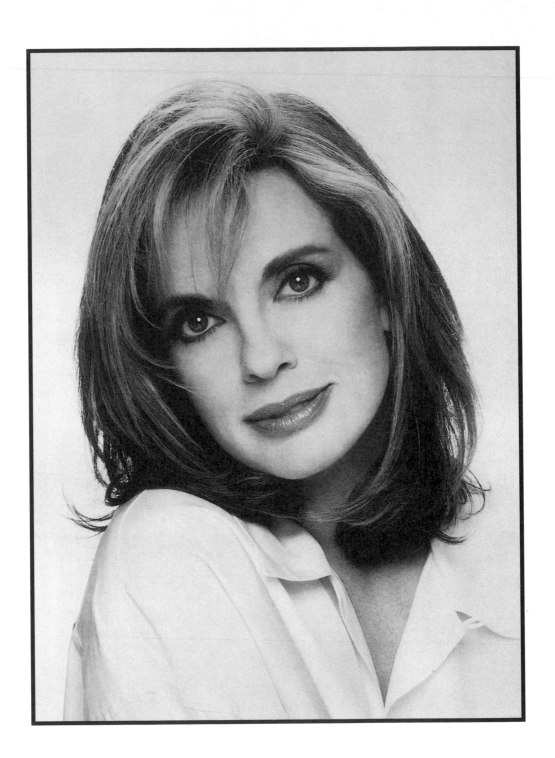

LINDA GRAY
ACTRESS

BORN
Santa Monica, California

PROFESSIONAL AWARDS
Emmy nomination,
Best Actress, 1978: "Dallas"
Woman of the Year Award from
the Hollywood Radio and
Television Society

CAREER HIGHLIGHTS
TELEVISION
"Models Inc."
"Melrose Place"
"All That Glitters"
"Marcus Welby, M.D."
"Broken Pledges: The Eileen
Stevens Story"
"Why My Daughter:
The Gayle Moffit Story"
"Return to Bonanza"
"Highway Casanova"

2 AYURVEDIC MEDICINE

"I left the clinic with a profound awareness of the role peace, harmony, and tranquility played in my health," Linda says. *"All I had learned about using ayurvedic medicine in my life seemed so intelligent. I resonated to it. It addressed all the ways my being could be out of sync and stressed, and how I needed to take time for myself every day."*

If you're lucky enough to get invited to a dinner party at Linda Gray's canyon home, break out your work boots and leave your fancy duds at home. Because sometime before you sit down to dinner, Linda will more than likely lead you and her caravan of guests into the organic vegetable and herb garden, where you'll choose your meal for the night.

Not quite what you'd expect from the queen of night-time soaps, is it?

But as Linda assures you, "it's quite an experience. I bless everything we eat, and with what remains, I make my own compost to recycle back into the earth."

As you might have guessed, eating in the Gray home is a sacred experience, where a vegetarian meal is more likely to appear on the table than heavy meats. Linda, with a calmness and serenity that bespeaks a deeply centered woman, believes that the food you put into your body, the way you prepare it, and with whom you choose to break bread are all critical to maintaining good health.

Considering that Linda looks better today than she did fifteen years ago, when she first achieved fame as Sue Ellen on the phenomenally successful TV series "Dallas," who could argue?

For Linda, the transformation began on "Dallas." While millions of viewers around the world tuned in each week to see what the sometimes naughty and always fashionable Sue Ellen was up to, it was an exhausted Linda who dragged herself home from the set each day.

Working what felt like twenty-hour days, Linda wondered how long she could keep it up before her stressed-out body simply collapsed. "I did what I could to stay balanced and healthy, but the truth is I was on total burnout," Linda says. "I tried to use whatever time I had off to pull myself together."

Besides acting, Linda also had kids to raise and a house to run.

"When we began shooting "Dallas," my kids were 11 and 13. When we finished, they were grown, and my daughter was married. They grew up on that set. Each year I had to uproot my entire family and move them down to Texas," then pack them up and return to Los Angeles a few months later.

"There was always so much work. And it was nonstop work that would go on for ten and a half months a year. Then, when we would finally go on hiatus, I would be asked to travel and promote the show in places like Australia and Europe."

For eleven straight years, Linda kept up this hectic pace.

"I did what I could to stay balanced," Linda says. "I was grabbing at things"—meditation and yoga, for instance—"to keep me there." This kept Linda going until she hit a particularly taxing year. "It had been one of those years from God-knows-where," says the actress. "We had just concluded another grueling year of filming, my daughter got married in India, and I finished directing a show.

"I was fried! I knew staying balanced and centered most of the time would get me through. But, at this point in my life, I just didn't know how."

Fortunately for Linda, a concerned and caring friend reached out and made a suggestion that would change Linda's life. "It seemed he had gone to this mind/body clinic in California, and his entire time there was about releasing stress," Linda remembers. "I happened to be on hiatus from the show, so I immediately picked up the phone and booked myself in for a week's stay."

Not knowing what to expect, except hopefully some relief from her stressed-out life, Linda arrived at the clinic, which at that time was located in Lancaster, California.

"When I got there, I didn't want to see anybody, be with anybody, or talk to anybody," says Linda. "I was led to a beautiful room in which I immediately felt comfortable. It was simple with this very clean feeling to it. And all I wanted to do was hang out there."

But Deepak Chopra, M.D., the famous author and celebrated doctor who ran the clinic, had another plan in mind. It included a full week of ayurvedic treatments designed to revive a stressed-out Linda and teach her how to cope with stress when she returned to her everyday life.

Dr. Chopra's approach is rooted in ayurveda, a 5,000-year-old system of medicine that emphasizes prevention over cure. It is based on the belief that the mind exerts the deepest control over the body and its health.

In ayurveda, health is defined as a state of balance and harmony among body, mind, and spirit.

Using centuries-old natural therapies, an individual treatment plan is designed for each patient according to their *dosha*, a metabolic "type" based on a number of physical and psychological traits.

Linda's first step was a comprehensive personal evaluation in which her habits and lifestyle were closely evaluated and her *dosha* defined. There are three *doshas*: *vata, pitta,* and *kapha.* Often a *dosha* is a combination of two metabolic types, the first being more prominent than the second, so that an individualized program of treatments can be designed.

Linda was told that her metabolic body type was *vata-pitta*. "It was explained to me with a cute little story," Linda says. "If you had airline tickets and were going away for a holiday, and you came up to the counter and were told that your flight had been canceled, the *vata*, which is me, would run over to another airline counter and say, 'All right, get me on your next plane out, I need to go.' The *pitta* would stand there and pound their fists and yell at the poor counter person who made the announcement, while the *kapha* would kind of saunter over to the ice-cream counter and say, 'We'll think about what to do.'

"I have a combined body type," adds Linda, "so for me it's like, 'Okay, plane canceled, change plans, let's go.' I'd be a little bit angry, but I probably wouldn't pound my fists.

"Now, that's a very simplistic way to explain the three body types. But when I heard the airport story about each of the body types it allowed me and everyone else who heard the story to see where they fit in." In ayurveda, your individual body type determines how your path to better health should be approached.

But even though this explanation of body types intrigued Linda, she preferred to stay in her room.

"I thought it would be so wonderful to just sleep in and meditate and do yoga," Linda recalls. "I thought, 'I'll get some rest, that will help revitalize me.'"

And it would. But while sleep, yoga, and meditation are treatments used in ayurveda, Dr. Chopra and the staff at the clinic had a lot more in mind for Linda to bring her back to maximum health.

"Deepak was concerned about me," says Linda. "He said, 'You'd better come down to have dinner with us.' But I told him I didn't want to see anybody. The last thing I wanted to be was charming or to put makeup on or, for that matter, do anything at all."

Dr. Chopra relented, and Linda compromised. The staff brought Linda's meals to her room, and when it was time for her specific treatment program, Linda went downstairs.

There was a lot in store for a still stressed-out Linda. She was about to be introduced to *panchakarma*, a collection of therapies all designed to rejuvenate and purify the body. This is done through the cleansing of the body and removal of "toxins," which in ayurveda are considered the root of disease.

"The clinic was housed in this beautiful mansion, and they would do all the treatments down in the basement," Linda says. "I became like this little mole, going down to the basement for treatments and right back up to my room as soon as they were finished."

Linda arrived in the basement for her first session of *panchakarma*. For the next two hours, Linda was treated to a very special massage and hot oil treatment. The herbalized oil massage is part of a soothing purification process designed to loosen impurities from the skin and stimulate the immune system.

All that was required of Linda was to lie back as her body revitalized itself to be awakened to its own "inner healer."

"But, nothing was more blissful, and I do mean bliss-full. Two women massaged my body in complete synchronicity, and I was moved into this euphoric state. It really balances your body. It's not like there is one person working on your ankle and somebody else on your shoulder. One does your left shoulder and one does your right, and they work your entire body this way. You lay back and close your eyes. They close their eyes too, but they still manage to work in perfect unison with each other to perform the massage.

"It made me very conscious of my body," Linda admits. "You also listen to some lovely music. It's all very soothing."

Once the massage was finished, the clinic staff drip hot sesame oil on you, Linda says. "It felt just wonderful. In fact, although they didn't recommend it, I kept it in all week. You are still lying down, but covered and with your head tilted back a little. They put this stainless steel bowl under your head and then drip warm oil on your forehead. It's not messy, it just sort of goes back onto your head, like a shampoo, after it hits your forehead. They use this plastic tubing like a funnel so that it doesn't get in your eyes, and they can direct its flow."

While having hot oil dripped on your face might be a little unnerving to some, Linda had quite a different reaction.

"It's this incredible feeling, sort of like going back to the womb," she says. "After my first treatments, I became so relaxed that I fell asleep. I would wake up and laugh with the therapists, asking them how long I was out. It got so that I would arrive for a treatment, and we would joke about how long it would take for me to fall asleep.

"You feel as if stress is being removed from the innermost portions of your being," Linda adds, "stress that you didn't even know you had.

"The stress felt like it was being released on a cellular level, and that it had been in my body for a very long time," says Linda. "It's the kind that just doesn't get released through napping or sleep, but instead gets deposited in the body. Then we drink coffee or another stimulant to mask it.

"But the oil treatment told my stress it's okay to come out of my body, and it felt like it was actually rising out of me."

LEARNING TO CREATE A STRESS-FREE LIFE

With all remaining stress wiped out of her body, Linda eagerly followed the program prescribed for her during the rest of her stay.

"Between treatments, I would stay in my room and read or watch the videos they provided to explain more about ayurvedic medicine," Linda says. "I'd take long baths and slip in some aromatherapy here and there. All the while, I had this beautiful music playing, which seemed to soothe another part of me. They gave me this aroma holder, which I would fill with an oil made specifically for my body type—*vata*—and I would also burn some incense.

"Every once in a while I would think to myself, 'Maybe I'll go into town and browse,' but I would end up staying in my room. Inside, I would hear my body calling for 'More! More! More!'"

Between treatments, Linda was shown how she could achieve maximum health with a specific diet and exercise plan, and how lifestyle choices made in alignment with her body type could help maintain a balance and harmony that would create maximum health.

In ayurveda, the types of food you eat, the thoughts you hold in your mind, the movements you do, and even the seasons and times of the day are thought to affect health.

"I really liked being given all this information on how I could best work with my body," Linda says. "It taught me how to have greater respect for my body.

"For my body type, I am not supposed to have anything that is cold. Our bodies thrive on warm, nurturing food like steamed vegetables and rice."

For Linda, who always ate what she considered a healthy diet, this would be quite a change. "I was always a cold salad and ice tea person," says the actress. "I had eaten this [way] to watch my weight."

Linda gave the new diet a try.

As for the exercise, "I liked doing yoga, which I've done on and off for years. I was never able to attend classes, given my work schedule, since most gyms don't open until 6 A.M. My work had me up at 4 A.M., so I learned to do it on my own."

Once Linda returned home from the clinic, she tried to retain the basic stress-reducing and body-enhancing strategies she'd learned. She stayed on her diet, continued with yoga, and meditated regularly. "I left the clinic with a profound awareness of the role peace, harmony, and tranquility played in my health," Linda says. "All I had learned about using ayurvedic medicine in my life seemed so intelligent. I resonated to it. It addressed all the ways my being could be out of sync and stressed, and how I needed to take time for myself every day."

But now that she was home from the clinic, how much of this would actually transfer over to Linda's busy and demanding life? A special diet while you're on a retreat is one thing, but how about when you're a busy actress always on the run?

"I found not having cold foods in the summer can be rough," says Linda. "I still wanted an ice tea or cold salad, but I have come to see that I do so much better with steamed vegetables and rice. My digestion is so much better. Now when I'm out at a restaurant and they serve ice water, I ask for room-temperature or even warm water."

Her digestion is also better because, in keeping with ayurvedic principles, she refuses to eat in a stressful situation. As a result, business appointments for breakfast, lunch, or dinner are a thing of the past.

"So much of ayurvedic medicine is a commonsense philosophy," says the actress. "If I'm out at a business meal, I get really distracted in terms of my eating and I may be in a hurry rather than honoring the food that I'm putting into my body. This doesn't work for me. Now I try never to have a meal with anyone in a business situation. When people say, 'Let's go out for dinner or lunch to talk business,' I don't go. I've come to see that my food doesn't digest well when I'm talking about business during a meal.

"I first discovered this at breakfast meetings, where everybody is so rushed having to get to the office. Then you have waiters interrupting you and nine people coming over to say hello. It made me nuts. I said, 'Okay, I'll try giving up breakfast meetings and see how that affects my work.' And it worked just fine. Then I took it a step further and said, 'No business meals, period.' And that works even better!"

A RETURN TO THE GARDEN

As a result of her experience with ayurveda, Linda pays particular attention to what's necessary in her life to stay stress-free. "It can be so difficult, especially for women who are balancing family, job, and children in the nineties," says Linda. That's why "I've tried to live very simply."

Linda took this path when she decided to remodel her home, which is known to be one of the most stress-filled experiences. "I was married to an art director, and we had a very lovely home," Linda explains. "When we got divorced, I ended up keeping it. But it was very dark, in a seventies style, and had a somewhat oppressive feeling.

"I ended up ripping everything out and painting everything white. I put huge cream tiles on the floors and added strong, feminine, light-colored furniture. I even added a Japanese fish pond so I can hear the water and feel the tranquility that it brought me.

"At some point, I began to see that what I was doing through the remodeling was creating an outward manifestation of who I had become and how healing this was for me."

Linda also kept up her meditation, a key component to ayurveda. "I find that when my life is fullest, and I think I can't fit one more thing into my day, that's when I value meditation and the effects it brings the most. We all get so busy thinking and running and buying this and that. But when I stop and take the time for meditation and simply being alone with myself, the world becomes a much happier and more peaceful place."

Ayurveda has also been good for her career, she acknowledges. "Meditation has allowed me to become much more intuitive and in touch with things that would otherwise pass me by," Linda says. "It even helped me get my role on 'Models Inc.,' Linda recalls, referring to a TV series in which she starred.

"I happened to be sitting in an office waiting to pick up my daughter, when I leafed through a magazine that was there. Wedged in between ten other articles was a small story on Aaron Spelling, creator of 'Dallas' and 'Melrose Place.' He was talking about the latest series he was about to produce, 'Models Inc.' He talked about the four women who were up for the lead—Raquel Welch, Angie Dickinson, Lauren Hutton, and Linda Evans. But I immediately knew that that was my role. I called my agent, and shortly thereafter I was offered the part."

There's nothing psychic involved, Linda says. "I found that with meditation, things like your level of intuition develop very quickly and you become better able to see things because you're more in balance, less stressed, and things feel simpler. You also have more energy available to act on these intuitive hits that seem to come across our plate all the time."

How often does she meditate? Twice a day for twenty minutes each time, usually in the morning and at night, says Linda. "That was recommended to me at the ayurveda clinic," Linda says. "With my schedule and never knowing what I am doing from one day to the next, I've learned to be very creative about how I fit this in. Sometimes I just get five minutes, but I don't beat myself up saying, 'Oh my God, I didn't get a full twenty.' And the nice thing about meditation is that you can do it just about anywhere. I find a comfortable chair and place my hands in my lap, and for twenty minutes I let my mind go of any extraneous thoughts and focus on nothing."

After a morning meditation, Linda follows through with the ayurvedic practice of applying oil to her body.

"The oil helps prepare my body for the day," says the actress. "It's very centering for me. It's also a special time I take just for me for self-nurturing. It's the way I say thank you to my body for doing all these nice things for me.

"First I heat the oil. Some people put it in the microwave, but I don't like going all the way to the kitchen. It's too cold and dark [at] that time of the morning, so I heat it in hot water. Then I pour it into my hands, and I rub it on my palms. I rub the top of my head with it for a few seconds, and then I go around to all the joints of my body in long movements. I brush around my elbows and shoulders. Everywhere there's a joint. I go over my whole body this way. Then I sit down and do the soles of my feet.

"If I'm in a real hurry, I'll just rub it on my face, hair, neck, and the soles of my feet. I'll also do my wrists and hands—all the key points.

"Sometimes I don't even have time to heat it up, so I use it at room temperature. The point is I try to do whatever I can, given my schedule, and when I have more time, I take it.

"When it's over, I feel like I've prepared my body for a more balanced day by taking the time for me and putting on this suit of oil, like armor. Rather than meditating and jumping into the shower, I do this to prepare my body for the day."

Although Linda has used ayurveda for eight years, she still returns to the Mind/Body Clinic—now in La Jolla, California—whenever she can find a chance.

"This year I've been there twice," Linda says. "I'm not saying that I follow everything 100 percent all the time. Every so often I reach for a cappuccino or don't make time for meditation.

"But I try to do things like drink my little *vata* tea, made especially for my body type and which I find very pacifying," she says. "It keeps me balanced, especially at times when I would tend to stress out."

Being back in a demanding television series certainly provides Linda with ample opportunities to test this out. While she makes no claim that her somewhat hyper *vata-pitta* body is completely stress-free, she does admit that when she practices ayurveda, things seem to be far more balanced than they have in the past.

So if you do manage to get invited to dinner at Linda's and notice the serenity that Linda radiates from head to toe, you'll know how it got there. As Linda freely admits, ayurveda "really works for me."

SPOTLIGHT ON AYURVEDA

Imagine arriving at the doctor's office for an initial consultation, only to be asked if your hair is naturally straight or wavy? Or if, on an average day, you tend to be calm or feisty?

You'd probably think you'd stumbled into a dating service rather than a doctor's office, but these are the types of questions that you'll be asked when you first visit an ayurvedic physician, an individual who synthesizes 5,000 years of folk medicine from India and applies it to your particular problems.

It's all part of determining your specific *dosha*, or metabolic body type. That's where all treatment begins in ayurvedic medicine. The goal is to figure out each patient's physical and psychological traits, then classify them into one of three general types: *vata*, an enthusiastic person with a restless mind who is usually a little on the thin side; *pitta*, an individual who is neat and smart with a touch of temper and a few bulges of muscle; or *kapha*, a calm, sweet person with a tendency to gain weight easily.

Individuals are asked about lifestyle, work habits, exercise regimens, emotional mood swings, and whether they tend to be light or heavy sleepers, quick risers, or slow to waken. All the while, they're observed: What color and makeup is the skin? How does it compare in color to others of the same race? Is the hair thick and wavy or thin and straight? Finally, the pulse is taken in twelve different places, and the tongue, eyes, and nails are examined. A urine sample is smelled and checked for color and clarity.

While it all may seem a bit labored, this initial consultation is viewed as crucial to treatment in this ancient form of health care. To an ayurvedic physician, treating a patient before knowing a body type is like a mechanic trying to fix an engine prior to knowing what kind of machine it is intended to power. You may get rid of the symptoms—loud crunching sounds, slow-moving parts—but it will never achieve maximum working order.

By the end of your initial exam, the ayurvedic doctor will classify you into one of the three metabolic body types. While it is common to be a combination of two or more of these *doshas*, there is generally one that is more prominent than another.

Once labeled, the patient is ready for a specific treatment program composed of many ancient healing techniques all designed to bring body, mind, and spirit into a state of balance—the Eastern definition of health. Ayurvedic physicians believe disease is caused by an imbalance of movement, structure, and metabolism. This is corrected by bringing the mind, body, and soul back into balance. The way to do this is to use specific techniques that have been custom-tailored to each of the three *doshas*.

From weight loss to hair loss, cancer prevention to treatment, colds to constipation, based on tradition and patient success stories, ayurvedic professionals claim almost any condition can be avoided or successfully treated through a program of yoga, meditation, diet, music, aromatherapy, herbal remedies, and *panchakarma*, a purification treatment that uses massage, healing oils, and enemas to balance the body and rid it of impurities.

Although there is an increasing body of evidence indicating that meditation is such an effective stress reliever that it can help lower blood pressure, evidence for any of the other ayurvedic practices is hard to come by. Ayurveda is not, however, short of personal endorsements. Billie Jean King, Martina Navratilova, Lindsay Wagner, and Alana Stuart Hamilton are but a few celebrities who have enjoyed the benefits of ayurveda.

Most ayurvedic practices combine folklore and common sense. Dietary recommendations, for example, are designed to enhance healthful digestion and balance the predominant *dosha* that exists within each of us. In ayurvedic tradition, the properties of each food are determined by its taste—whether it is sweet, sour, salty, bitter, pungent, or astringent. The effects of that food on digestion are generally characterized as heavy or light, moist or dry, cold, cooling, warm, or hot.

Depending on your body type, you will be advised to either emphasize or eliminate certain tastes in cooking to balance your system. If you are a *kapha* who has asthma, for instance, your doctor might recommend pungent spices like pepper, which breaks up the mucus and congestion commonly found in *kaphas*. But the same seasoning, while perfect for a *kapha*, can have the opposite effect on a *pitta*—producing heartburn and irritability.

While there are some foods that work for all three *doshas*, in times of illness doctors will recommend foods specifically designed to bring greater balance to the specific body type.

There is also a group of underlying nutritional principles that apply to all three body types. These principles include eating only when seated in a soothing place and eating only when you are hungry. They also dictate that you should never eat when you are upset, nor should you eat too rapidly or too slowly. Waiting two to four hours between meals, never talking with your mouth full, and never eating in bed are thought to play a part in keeping the body balanced.

Up until approximately twenty years ago, ayurveda was relatively unknown in Western countries until the former chief of staff at New England Memorial Hospital, Deepak Chopra, M.D., first popularized what he believed were the extraordinary healing powers of this ancient form of health care. Trained in Western medicine at India's most prestigious medical school, Dr. Chopra soon abandoned his mainstream position to become the voice of ayurveda.

For the past ten years, Dr. Chopra has lectured, taught, and promoted ayurveda until he has almost single-handedly established a large Western audience. He also has created a large audience for his own books and tapes along the way. Today, Dr. Chopra's books have sold more than three million copies, and he has appeared on influential talk shows such as "Oprah."

Want to give ayurveda a try? First, find your specific body type. Try reading one of Dr. Chopra's best-sellers, and you'll find quizzes that will help you figure it out, plus details of ayurvedic practices you can learn on your own.

Here's one simple practice you *can* do at home—meditation. Begin by setting aside a few minutes to be alone—no kids, no TV. Sit down in a comfortable chair, but resist lying back. You might fall asleep! Relax your shoulders by shrugging them a few times. Then let your head fall forward with your chin nearly touching your chest, and move your head slowly from side to side. Lift your head erect again and close your eyes. Start to relax by following your breath with your mind. B-r-e-a-t-h-e *in* relaxation, breathe *out* worries and concerns. Breathe in through your nose, slowly counting to five. Slowly exhale each time. Try to empty your mind of your everyday thoughts. If you find your mind starting to wander off to the pile of laundry or to a phone call you have to make, call to mind a pleasant memory or picture you may have seen—ocean waves as they meet the beach, a sunset in the mountains, or a sunrise over a misty lake—and breathe deeply again. How do you feel now? This should give you a feel for this ancient healing art. But for the real thing, you'll want to learn from a trained meditation teacher.

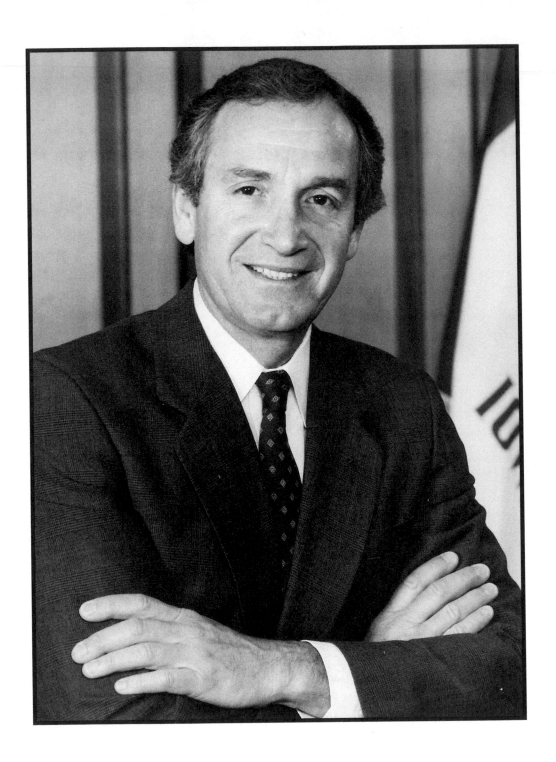

3 BEE POLLEN THERAPY

BORN
November 19, 1939,
Cumming, Iowa

EDUCATION
B.A., Iowa State University
L.L.B., Catholic University of
America Law School

CAREER HIGHLIGHTS
Elected to U.S. Senate,
1984–present
Elected to U.S. House of
Representatives, 1974–1984
Initiated legislation to create
the Office of Alternative
Medicine with the National
Institutes of Health

"If people would just take the time to stop and think about their health, they would know more deep down inside about what is happening to their bodies than the doctors who examine them. It's common sense."

Sitting in an oak-paneled hearing room in the United States Senate Office Building in Washington, D.C., Tom Harkin, a senator from Iowa, settled into a high-backed chair to wait for his invited guests—the esteemed members of the United States Senate and their staffs.

On the table in front of him were sample tablets of bee pollen. Beside him was Royden Brown, the seventy-something author of the *Bee Hive Product Bible*.

The senator, as he later explained, was hosting this unusual party to demonstrate the fact that there are low-cost alternatives to the budget-busting traditional health-care treatments both the government and individual consumers are asked to pay for every year. The party was a great success.

Not only did at least a few of the Senate's distinguished members find relief from their allergies, but the entire Congress, at Senator Harkin's behest, subsequently appropriated $2 million to launch the Office of Alternative Medicine within the National Institutes of Health to investigate, through controlled scientific studies, whether or not nontraditional therapies like bee pollen could actually offer an alternative to the high cost of staying healthy in America.

What could lead a Washington insider to consider the legitimacy of alternative healing?

It was former Representative Berkley Bedell who first got Harkin interested in alternative health care. Bedell, who entered the United States House of Representatives the same year—1974—as Harkin, is a man the senator holds in high regard. "Here's a guy who's close to seventy years old and in Congress," says Harkin. "But he came down with Lyme disease and prostate cancer. Not one, but both at once. He was forced to quit Congress."

Unfortunately for Bedell, at that time, not may doctors were familiar with the diagnosis or treatment of Lyme disease. Although we now know that antibiotics can cure Lyme disease if caught in the early stages, the doctors were unable to cure his condition. "He was forced to look outside the medical community," says Harkin. "And after searching for a while, he found in Canada a highly unconventional but nonetheless effective cure for his Lyme disease," using whey made from cow colostrum, the first milk of a cow that has just given birth.

Bedell's prostate cancer also forced him to seek out nontraditional therapies, adds Harkin. That's because Bedell had an operation to remove prostate cancer, but the surgeons were unable to get it all. "I remember telling my wife, 'He looks like death warmed over,' " says Harkin, shaking his head. "But Berkley was not one to give up. He continued his search for an alternative cure—and found it in Canada. It's been six or seven years since then, and there are no traces of cancer."

Congressman Bedell's results were enough to make him a staunch believer in alternative medicine. But when he tried to share the good news with the Washington scientific establishment, asking them to investigate other alternatives to traditional medicine, he was ignored.

Bedell turned to Senator Harkin.

"He came to me frustrated that he couldn't get the National Institutes of Health to listen. Because he's not a doctor, they ignored his claims about how he was cured. But eventually I got the Office of Alternative Medicine set up and funded."

CHERRY BLOSSOM TIME

During the spring of 1993, Senator Harkin found himself smack in the middle of pollen season, sneezing and sniffling his way through a meeting with Berkley Bedell.

Cherry blossom time, Washington's unofficial pronouncement that spring has arrived, might be one of the most beautiful times of the year to be in our nation's capital, but for an allergy sufferer it's also the most aggravating.

"Over the years my allergies had become progressively worse—especially during the spring and fall allergy seasons," says Harkin. "My doctor had prescribed a mild antihistamine, one that I had been taking for years. When it no longer worked, I went back to my doctor, and he prescribed a more powerful dose. That worked for another year or so. But finally it didn't work any longer, either."

So with his antihistamine no longer effective and cherry blossom time about to begin in Washington once again, Harkin started using over-the-counter cold and allergy capsules. "But they really weren't helping much," says the senator. "Even after taking them, I would still wake up in the middle of the night with these horrible sneezing fits, unable to breathe. I was driving my wife nuts."

Witnessing his friend sneezing his way through the people's business every day, Congressman Bedell made a suggestion. "Berkley told me he had a friend who claimed he could get rid of any allergy with bee pollen," says Harkin. "He asked if I would be interested in seeing him."

Harkin said yes. "I was introduced to Royden Brown. He came to my office, and we talked about bee pollen and what he thought it could do for me. He was very enthusiastic."

Brown brought several bottles of bee pollen with him that day. "When I looked at the bottles and read the ingredients, I saw that it contained other things besides bee pollen," says Harkin. "And I immediately realized that I was allergic to just about everything contained in the tablets."

Although Senator Harkin was aware that deliberately taking something to which he was allergic could cause his airway to swell and shut down his breathing, he approached the matter cautiously and decided to give the bee pollen a try.

"First, I was told to take a little and put it under my tongue to see if I had any reaction to it," says Harkin. After a few minutes, no swelling, redness, or itchiness had appeared anywhere. Harkin decided it was time to take his first dose.

"I was instructed to take what seemed like a massive dose, twelve of the tablets with water," Harkin recalls. "Then I was to wait a few minutes, about ten, to see if any of my symptoms were clearing up. I was told that if after the initial dose of twelve, there was no relief, I should take twelve more and continue doing this at measured intervals until I saw my symptoms clear up. That would be my signal to stop."

That was a good day to test the bee pollen remedy, since Harkin was having a particularly difficult time coping with his allergies. "That morning I had come to work with both eyes kind of puffy and red—you know how you feel when you have allergies.

"I thought it was kind of wild, but okay. That morning I took twelve tablets and then twelve more. I thought a little while later, 'Maybe my eyes are getting a little better, they seem to itch less.' But I thought, 'No, that's just psychological stuff.'"

The next day, he persevered with the treatment. "I took twelve tablets, then twelve more. I started writing down how many of them I was taking. Finally, on the third day, I took sixty of them.

"It made me a little sick to my stomach, so I called Mr. Brown. He told me to lay off the bee pollen for a few days, but I kept taking it anyway."

Why on earth would he keep taking something that seemed to make him sick?

"People can do a lot to take care of themselves," replies Harkin. "I feel very strongly about that. If people would just take the time to stop and think about their health, they would know more deep down inside about what is happening to their bodies than the doctors who examine them. It's basically common sense." Despite the mild reaction, he decided to trust the process.

Harkin left Washington a few days later to attend a political retreat. He continued taking the bee pollen, all the while wondering when it was going to do something.

"When I got home from the retreat," says the senator, "I realized my allergies had left. No tapering off, they just left. This was about the sixth day. My eyes had cleared up, my nose had cleared up, and I wasn't sneezing."

When he realized his allergies had simply disappeared, the senator called Brown to let him know how well the bee pollen had worked. "He was very matter-of-fact about it," says Harkin. "He said, 'I knew it would help clear up your allergies.'"

But when Harkin made the same announcement to members of the medical establishment, he received a different response. "I had doctors tell me that the bee pollen is nonsense," says the senator. "But all I can say is, 'I'm sorry. Something happened when I took the bee pollen. I know what I was like before, and I know what I was like after taking it, so please don't tell me it didn't happen.' Of course it did, and I've been taking bee pollen ever since."

Every day Senator Harkin takes six tablets of bee pollen as a preventive measure. "At the start of the spring and fall pollen seasons, I usually take an additional dose of raw bee pollen," he adds. "I have it in addition to my usual tablets. At those times of year, I generally take tablets in the middle of the day as well. And I take it whenever any of my allergy symptoms start to flare up. I think the secret is to get over a certain point, then keep it up. I think what most people do with alternative medicine is that they want that cold pill to work in one hour for a quick fix. They don't understand that you have to use it over a period of time. People give up on it too easily.

"I must admit that sometimes, especially in the spring, I still feel my allergies coming on," says Harkin. "But it's nothing like it was before. I no longer have sneezing fits, my eyes don't get puffy, and I don't get all clogged up. I simply take some bee pollen, and the symptoms stop."

This type of low-cost, nontoxic health care clearly appeals to Harkin as a policymaker as well as a consumer. "I think there is a tremendous cry in this country for a health-care system," says the senator. "What we have is a sick-care system. 'If you get sick, we'll take care of you.' But people want to try things to keep themselves healthy in the first place. They want to build up their bodies, and they want to get away from toxic drugs."

Gesturing to a photo in his office of a single man trying to stop the Chinese political establishment by lying down in front of a tank in Tiananmen Square, Senator Harkin explains that knowing how people feel is why he's metaphorically laid himself down in front of the American medical establishment in Washington. "We have a National Institute of Allergy and Infectious Diseases that has never looked at bee pollen in a controlled scientific study," says the senator. "I want them to look at it. They think it's hokum. But I want them to work in the future to help substantiate some of the claims about [those] alternative health treatments that work—and weed out the quacks who are busy selling snake oil."

SPOTLIGHT ON BEE POLLEN

Have an allergy? Need to lose weight, build muscle, or erase wrinkles?

Bee pollen, billed as "nature's perfect and complete food" by its advertisers, is touted as a cure for allergies, impotence, obesity, underdeveloped muscles, wrinkles, insomnia, respiratory conditions, digestive disorders, sore throats, and tired kidneys.

There's no scientific evidence to back up these claims, of course, although honey itself does have some antibacterial properties. But that hasn't stopped one in every five Americans from trying this supplement in one form or another—including former President Ronald Reagan, whose youthful countenance despite the ravages of Alzheimer's disease is legendary.

Just where does bee pollen come from? It's made from the pollen gathered by bees from the male center of a flower. Honeybees visit the flowers and carry pollen back to their hives as food for their own colony. We then rely on experienced beekeepers to extract it from the honeycombs.

While used by many as a food supplement for an added nutritional punch, the most common use of bee pollen is in treating allergies. By administering small amounts of the pollen—generally in tablet form—proponents claim that you can stimulate the immune system and make the allergy sufferer produce antibodies to the pollen. The result? The allergies stop. If you're allergic to pollen, never use bee pollen products without first consulting your doctor. Your immune system may produce a life-threatening reaction.

If you do decide to try it, don't worry about having to don a beekeeper's mask or reach into a hive to use it. There are so many people buzzing around singing the praises of this natural product that it is commonly sold in drug and health food stores around the world.

The mystique surrounding bee pollen probably accounts for its popularity as much as testimonials that it cures everything from cancer to warts. For centuries, ancient cultures have been extolling its virtues. The Bible, Talmud, and Koran all include glowing reports of its use. Hippocrates, the father of modern medicine, was among the first to prescribe this magic elixir, claiming its "warmth" could cure a host of common complaints including sores and ulcers. In ancient Athens and Greece, athletes who wanted to improve their endurance and stamina often turned to bee pollen as a dietary supplement.

Today, athletes turn to this food for added energy and strength. As a beauty product, whether taken internally as a daily supplement or used externally as part of a prepared cream, it is thought to enhance the skin due to its rejuvenating properties and is helpful in treating skin sores and acne. At ninety calories per one-ounce serving, it is also being sold as a dietary supplement for weight loss.

Perhaps no group has become as enamored with its claims of rejuvenation as the geriatric crowd, who have been told by advertisers that it's a real fountain of youth. Believers claim it is a natural remedy for old age and, when taken in daily doses, will increase memory and concentration while strengthening the cardiovascular and respiratory systems.

No discussion of the healing power of this mystical substance could be complete without talking about its use as a sexual stimulant. Whether as an adjunct cure to impotency or to help with sexual endurance, bee pollen has gotten quite a reputation in this area.

While modern producers have unsuccessfully tried to create an artificial substance to resemble natural bee pollen, there is only one real source for bee pollen: the bees themselves. It is available in many forms: fresh, canned, and in tablets or capsules. Used like vitamins to enhance the nutritional value of many foods, bee pollen is also finding its way into many common products such as cereal and drinks.

If you decide to give it a try, consider adding it to your cereal as a topping, sprinkling it on your salad, or slipping some into your morning fruit juice. Its sweet taste is barely noticeable.

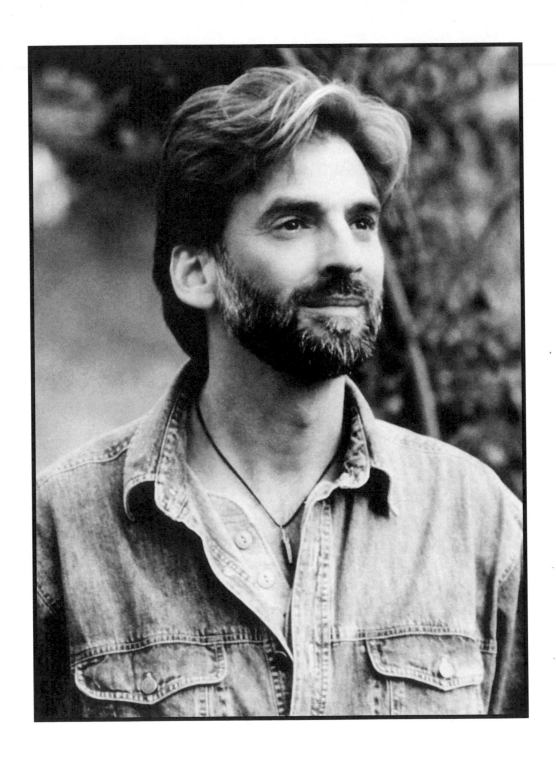

4 COLON HYDROTHERAPY

BORN
January 7, 1948,
Everett, Washington

PROFESSIONAL AWARDS
Academy Award nomination,
1981: "Footloose"
Cable Ace Award and two Emmy
Awards, 1994: TV special
"This Island Earth"
Grammy Award, 1981:
"What a Fool Believes" (writer)
Grammy Award, 1981:
"This Is It" (singer)

CAREER HIGHLIGHTS
1970–1976: member of
Loggins & Messina
1976–present: solo career

PLATINUM ALBUMS
Leap of Faith
Celebrate Me Home
Night Watch

GOLD ALBUMS
Return to Pooh Corner
Vox Humana

SINGLES
Over ten #1 singles

"I used colonics to help bring emotional clarity and get in touch with me."

Kenny Loggins knows what it's like to have the kind of feelings that come straight from your soul and let you know you're alive. He also knows how to take those feelings and turn them into words and music that touch our lives.

But there was a time when Kenny felt as if he was losing that inner connection—the key to his creativity. And while it wasn't apparent to his millions of fans, to Kenny, the signs were obvious. "If you look at the cover of *Back to Avalon*," says Kenny, commenting on the album he created during those tumultuous times, "you'll see a man in pain. It was one of the saddest times of my life."

It was a time in which he was questioning much about his life, his choices, his relationships, including whether or not the love he had shared in a fifteen-year marriage—a relationship that had produced three terrific kids and lots of happy times—was in fact "the real thing." Kenny felt emotionally stuck. So, pulled by no more than his intuition, Kenny decided to look inside himself for clarity and, he hoped, some answers.

"I've learned that as I listen to my intuition, I'm able to shift my life accordingly," Kenny explains. "I was looking for ways to connect with the spiritual parts of my life. I had a strong feeling that what I was putting into my body wasn't helping my frame of mind, so I wanted to clean it up and see what would happen.

"Most of this searching was unsure on my part," Kenny adds. "I never knew if I was going to get anywhere. I felt emotionally confused. But by cleaning out my body, I hoped I could change my relationship to myself and maybe from there, some sense of knowing and of healing would come from within."

Kenny had more than a need for healing. "When I get in touch with myself, that automatically gets me in touch with my creativity," says the song-writer. "My writing has been motivation for me to go inside and get a sense of what's going on. The carrot that gets dangled in front of me is that maybe a song will come from this." In fact, "all of the alternative healing I've used—chiropractic, acupuncture, diet, massage, and Rolfing—have been to clear the deadwood out of the way so that I could get in touch with *me*."

A RUSH OF WATER AND SOME VEGGIE BROTH

To meet his need for inner cleansing, Kenny turned to colon hydrotherapy, a procedure in which a trained technician uses a machine to flush the colon, or bowel, with water.

"It's exactly like any enema you might do at home," explains Julia Cooper, the Santa Barbara therapist who assisted Kenny, "except that it uses a small amount of pressure to clean out more of the bowel than a home enema might be able to reach."

"Julia shared an office in town with a homeopath and a therapist," Kenny says. "The room where she performed the colonics was small, sort of like a doctor's cubicle that she had fixed up to accommodate her work. I was sent to another room to get undressed," then given the choice of an open-back gown or towel. "I wrapped a towel around my waist and laid down on a table.

There are two positions that I was asked to move into during the treatment. One was lying down on my back with my knees in the air and my feet planted on the table under my knees; the other, lying on my side with my knees together brought up to about my waist, sort of what it would be like sleeping on your side with your knees curled up. In both positions, the towel was draped around me for modesty. But given the high level of intimacy involved with the colonic, it didn't really feel necessary. Then a tube with a specially designed disposable end was inserted. All I had to do was lie there and relax while the colon therapist did the rest. It didn't hurt. All I felt was the rush of the water. The session lasted a little longer than an hour."

During the initial session, Kenny discovered that Julia was well-versed in nutrition as well, so Kenny talked with her about a fast he wanted to do in conjunction with her therapy. This is not an unusual adjunct to colon therapy, so Julia recommended a vegetable juice fast that Kenny began the next day.

"I was heading for a week's stay in the high desert and decided to do it while I was there." The fast consisted of vegetable juice during the day with a hot vegetable broth at night. "It wasn't easy to stick to," Kenny admits. "By that evening, I got this headache over my right eye, and I felt nauseous. I thought it was something I had to tough through, but I found it so painful I said to myself that I'd do damn near anything to get rid of it."

Kenny called Julia to find out what he should do. "She asked me if I had done the enemas yet," he recalls. Of course, Kenny had forgotten. Julia had told him to give himself enemas during the fast because she believed that poisons in his organs would be dumped into his bloodstream and bowel—often causing physical discomfort, but easily dealt with. Although the body is naturally set up to eliminate everything in the bowel, Julia felt that enemas would help the process along and relieve any of the fasting's side effects, such as headaches and nausea.

Kenny had brought an enema bag with him, the kind you find in the local drugstore, and using nothing more than water, gave himself the enema. "It was the first time I had ever given myself anything like that, but it was really nothing, just like pouring water into your body, except from the other end," says the musician with a smile. Fortunately for Kenny, the enema took the headache away in less than fifteen minutes.

When Kenny returned from the desert he went to see Julia. "After the first colonic, I wasn't aware of anything much happening. But because of the way she helped me with the fast, there was a level of trust developing between us," Kenny says, "enough to pull me back to try more colonics."

Kenny signed on for a series of six colonics—one session a week for six weeks. After only a few sessions, Kenny was beginning to get some results. "I was starting to feel an overall glow," Kenny says. "It felt very cleansing, and I had a sense of elation, a sort of feeling of lightness that I had never before experienced. The truth is, eventually when you get off the table you feel pretty good."

Many practitioners feel that maximum benefits are derived when a person feels a connection with their colon hydrotherapist. "We would have these deep soul talks during the colonics," Kenny says. "Julia has a gentle quality that is so nurturing. I felt safe with her." And maybe that's why during the entire process Kenny felt as though he was cleansing himself both physically *and* emotionally.

"As a result, I found sadness, and I found joy," says Kenny. "But mostly I began to *feel* at a very deep level. The scary part of this is that you start to feel things that you haven't wanted to, as well as things that you do. But I had the willingness to see what was going on inside of me. I used colonics to help bring emotional clarity and get in touch with *me*."

Julia remembers Kenny's pain. "For many," Julia comments, "colonics is the most intimate experience of alternative health care they have ever had and in an area that is real scary for them, but most tend to move into a state of trust quickly. The more skill a colon therapist has in emotional issues the better, even if it is just conversation along with the colonics."

During the colonic sessions, Kenny found himself releasing angry feelings of the past both off and on the table. Old thought patterns and painful memories would surface during his discussions with Julia. After a few more sessions, Julia suggested he try some deep emotional release work she'd been trained in called the Fisher-Hoffman Process, a psychological technique that addresses family issues. (Julia's special training in this area is not common with colon hydrotherapists, nor is it part of the standard treatment.)

Kenny recalls, "As a result of the deep emotional work Julia was leading me through, I would sometimes get a headache over the right side of my head. There was so much being emotionally cleared at that time that we would go straight to the colonic table to remove the headache and nausea I was feeling.

"I know to some people this might seem like a pretty dramatic route to go just to get in touch with your feelings, but in fact I see it as a very basic and expeditious route. First off, it's the old 'your body being the temple of God' thing. And I just wanted to clean up the temple.

"For me it was all very simple: I had lost touch with my feelings, so I had to take the factors out of the way that might be blocking them. I also found that sugar and alcohol were the two primary things that emotionally numbed me. Whenever I would get really scared, I would unconsciously reach for something sweet that would insulate me or put an invisible wall around me. It created an emotional fog that wouldn't let anyone in, even the people who loved me. I could watch my walls go up. I try not to use sugar and alcohol anymore."

A NEW LIFE—AND WIFE

It's been 11 years since Kenny first began his colon hydrotherapy, and he has made many major changes in his life. Probably the most significant is that Julia is now his wife, and they are the adoring parents of young Lukas, their two-year-old son.

"When we first met, we were both married," Kenny admits. "But it wasn't until we were each separated that we began to view each other romantically. It was a beautiful irony. As I worked with Julia, I healed my life and became more capable of feeling it. I was able to see what was working and what wasn't working. I was able to respond. I also became more capable of being in a relationship with someone like Julia.

"But please understand," adds the songwriter. "My first marriage was by no means a mistake. We loved each other as best we could, for who we were at the time. Through our marriage, we both grew enough to eventually be able to set each other free."

Kenny and Julia work hard to maintain a "conscious" marriage—one where neither one supports each other's fears, and one in which both are encouraged to feel even all the things people are generally afraid to. "This kind of relationship takes you to some pretty scary places, especially the ones inside ourselves that we think are not lovable," says Kenny.

Since their marriage, Kenny has continued with colon hydrotherapy. "If I go through a particularly high period, let's say where Julia and I are feeling very connected and we have a couple of days of bliss, I seem to usually go into a detox right after that."

Translation? "The things we were taught about ourselves and life can show up in our bodies as places of tension or contraction. They'd simply have to let go for a while in order for me to love in that way," explains Kenny. "I guess that's how love heals. I can be totally open-hearted and as high as a kite from the love I am experiencing. That's when the old limiting consciousness literally starts to break loose and dumps toxins into my body. I often come out of that period with an intense headache. This is where colonic hydrotherapy comes in. Colonics are what I use to take away the pain."

It's a full and happy Loggins family temporarily occupying a beach house while they await renovation of a new home, which they hope will also give them a bit more privacy. "Having kids around from a toddler all the way up to a fourteen-year-old, there is always some kid after us," laughs Julia. Not that she's complaining. On the contrary, motherhood has made Julia bloom. Nevertheless, "when we can, we get away for a 'date night' at a local bed-and-breakfast," says Julia.

"All my work in alternative health has helped me, but I have a feeling that our love for each other has saved my life," says Kenny. "And that's what the work is all about. That's why you do colonics, diet, and emotional work—to love and be loved."

But Kenny recognizes that his choice is not for everyone. "With all of these alternative therapies, you have to believe that there is somewhere else better than where you are," says the musician. "You also have to know that you deserve to go there. It's all part of the process of trusting your inner voice enough to do something radical—to throw away the old forms and embrace something that speaks to you from an intuitive place, like colon therapy spoke to me.

"With so many forms of alternative therapy around, people have many different options available to them," adds Kenny. "Some they may read about and say 'That sounds interesting.' They may pass over all the rest. But there will be one that resonates for them, and that will be their pathway."

While checking out colon hydrotherapy might not bring you a hit album, an incredible relationship, and a baby boy, Kenny says, it just might clear the way—figuratively speaking, of course—to bring about some good changes in your own life.

SPOTLIGHT ON COLON HYDROTHERAPY

Colon hydrotherapy is one form of alternative therapy not likely to be discussed around the dinner table—unless you happen to be dining with one of many people who compare the experience to everything from a spiritual awakening to feeling, for the first time in their lives, clean and light inside.

The treatment itself is quite simple. The person receiving colonics lies on his back with his knees up and feet on the table. A colon hydrotherapist gently guides a tubelike applicator with a disposable tip called a speculum through the anus and into the first three inches of the rectum. Warm water under gentle pressure is then released through a two-way tube into the colon. One side of the tube irrigates the colon, using water to flush fecal matter from the body. This material is then released through the other half of the tube. The whole process, which takes about an hour, is not unlike an enema, except deeper cleansing occurs due to the amount of water being flushed through the machine.

The colon, which comprises the large intestine, anus, and rectum, is critical to the functioning of the entire digestive system. Uncoiled, it is five feet long and has many small pockets where it can store fecal matter that would be better off eliminated from the bodies. Fortunately, the body is designed so that fecal material is regularly and automatically moved through the colon by wavelike electrical contractions that are stimulated every time you put something in your mouth. That's why you frequently need to go to the bathroom after you eat.

But many colon hydrotherapists believe that everyone's colon is in some way impacted with fecal material. They believe that the inorganic chemicals found in the foods we eat and the air we breathe, plus drug residues and the remnants of illness, such as dead cells, all work to impact the colon. They also believe that anything people consume can get stored in the body—including bacteria, fungi, viruses, and parasites. If this situation is ignored, colonics therapists believe the body dumps these substances into the bloodstream, a process that plays havoc with the liver, lungs, and kidneys, and the circulatory, immune, and lymphatic systems.

Scientists acknowledge that bacteria, fungi, viruses, and parasites all can infect the body, but they do not support the concept that colonic hydrotherapy will aid in their removal from the body. Colonics *may*, scientists say, speed up the body's natural process of elimination. Clearly, the validity of colon hydrotherapy is an area of contention between mainstream thinkers and the hundreds of thousands of satisfied clients who continue to return to colon hydrotherapy for what they describe as its nurturing beneficial treatments.

Colon hydrotherapists believe there are times that colonics may be particularly helpful, such as when the body experiences stress or the individual tries to withdraw from an addictive habit such as smoking, alcohol, or even caffeine. They also believe it can help relieve a wide range of physical symptoms including bloating, backaches, fatigue, sinus conditions, bad breath, constipation, and even skin problems.

While emphasizing that the procedure is a service and not a medical treatment, colonic hydrotherapists generally recommend a series of sessions—one a week for six to ten weeks. Sessions are frequently preceded and followed by light diets of vegetable juices and broths. Side effects may include headaches, body aches, and nausea—all normal reactions that generally subside within a day. If these symptoms persist, you should contact your medical practitioner.

Colonics may have originated with the use of enemas in Egypt around 1500 B.C. The practice moved into what passed for mainstream medicine when Hippocrates, the father of medicine, recommended it for many common ailments that beset Greek society at the time. With the birth of naturopathic medicine in the late 1800s and early 1900s, colonics was touted as the ticket to good health, along with many other natural remedies. Colonic irrigators, the original machines used to administer colonics, became commonplace in doctors' offices and hospitals throughout the country in the 1920s and 1930s. They lost favor as the medical community questioned the value of the process and as pharmaceuticals were developed to treat some of the same symptoms that the irrigators had been treating. But since the 1970s, colonics has again emerged within the alternative therapy movement as a valued natural healing therapy.

If you decide to try colon hydrotherapy, you should choose a practitioner with whom you feel comfortable, given the intimate nature of contact. "Colon hydrotherapists are much like massage therapists in that the approach may differ from therapist to therapist," says Santa Barbara-based colon hydrotherapist Terry Allred. "How comfortable you feel with both the procedure and the person administering it can affect the value you receive from the therapy. A session can last up to one and a half hours, so choose wisely the person you are going to work with. If you feel uncomfortable during a session, tell the practitioner," she adds. "He or she is trained to understand your feelings and wants to make you as comfortable as possible."

One word of caution: Older folks, children, and anyone who may have a health problem should check with a doctor before undergoing colon hydrotherapy.

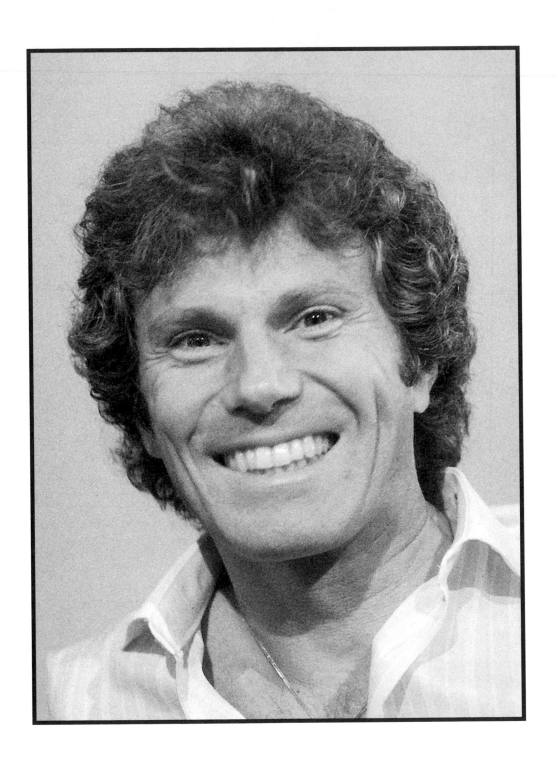

5 CREATIVE VISUALIZATION

BORN
October 12, 1942,
Hollywood, California

EDUCATION
B.S., economics,
Stanford University

CAREER HIGHLIGHTS
New Christy Minstrels,
founding member
Business consultant
Real estate developer
President of the
Wilderness Experience

AUTHOR
*The Writings of the Wall:
Peace at the Berlin Wall, 1990*

"I remember waking up and hearing this snap. It was like a rubber band breaking. When I tried to pull myself out of bed, I couldn't. My doctor told me there was a chance I'd never walk again."

Meet Terry Tillman.

Terry is a successful fifty-two-year-old businessman who formed a million-dollar real estate development company in California the year he graduated from Stanford. He's also a pilot, white-water rafting guide, runner, skier, author, and a founding member of the sixties folk group, The New Christy Minstrels.

Clearly Terry is a guy who grabs life with both hands and lives it in the fast lane. But there finally came a point when even he admits that his action-packed life was about to skid out of control.

"I was living on two hours of sleep a night and suffering from stress-induced insomnia," Terry explains as he relaxes between phone calls in his Santa Monica office.

"In those days, I had a steady diet of twelve cups of coffee a day, fast food, and three-martini dinners.

"I also consumed up to six aspirins a day," he adds. "That was to help with a headache I picked up one morning that lasted close to ten years. Given what I crammed into an average day, my guess is that it was stress-induced.

"The aspirins provided partial relief," says Terry, "but I was always aware of a dull ache."

It wasn't a healthy lifestyle, he acknowledges. And it was only a matter of time until his body let him know how it felt about the abuse.

ALONE IN IDAHO

When Terry's body decided to rebel, he was temporarily living in Idaho. "I had a few business interests there, including a magnificent house that wasn't selling," explains the entrepreneur. Terry had moved his base of operations to Idaho so he could focus on selling the house. He wasn't going to let it go without a fight—at least not until the morning he woke up, stretched, and heard something snap in his back.

"I actually heard the snap," says a still-amazed Terry. "And within seconds an unbearable pain overcame me."

Alone in the house with no one to help, Terry couldn't move. "I didn't get out of bed for the first twelve hours or so because every movement increased the pain, and I was afraid of doing permanent damage," explains Terry. "Eventually I either got numb or the pain subsided enough for me to pull myself across the bed to the phone."

A chiropractor from Ketchum arrived in response to Terry's call and suggested that Terry might have been flattened by a herniated, or slipped, disk. Since there was a possibility that he had damaged a nerve when the disk slipped, the chiropractor urged Terry to call an ambulance and get to the hospital for a CAT scan.

Although a slipped disk frequently heals on its own within two to six weeks, the chiropractor was concerned that damaged nerves might require surgery. But when Terry heard the word *surgery*, he refused to budge. "With surgery, no matter how successful, there was no guarantee I would be able to walk again, let alone run."

When it came down to it, the man who had lived life taking physical and financial risks didn't like the odds for this particular procedure. "I had spent years training for marathons, running, skiing, and rafting," explains Terry. "I loved being active. And the thought that I might have to give it up was devastating."

Terry looked for alternatives.

"I had taken a seminar in the mid-seventies that introduced me to the concept of creative visualization," he says. "I was told how powerful my thoughts were—how, by simply redirecting the energy I was using to create my financial success, I could produce great changes in my life."

Terry learned that creative visualization works on the premise that the world around us is composed of energy. He also learned that many people who practice creative visualization believe energy can be manipulated by thought. If you focus on the thought that you want to be rich and visualize yourself against a backdrop of affluence, for example, some adherents of creative visualization believe that you can literally program yourself to create greater wealth.

But does it work?

"During the seminar we were shown a creative visualization technique that involved using your imagination to heal a part of your body that was experiencing discomfort," says Terry. "For me it was easy to decide what I wanted to work on. You don't take eight aspirins a day" and not dream about relief. "So I thought, 'If I can get some relief from my headaches, I'd know there was something to this creative visualization stuff.'"

The seminar instructor told Terry to sit down and relax, then visualize a rose or even a pink elephant. Then once the instructor felt Terry and the other members of his group were in touch with their imaginations, he directed them to imagine specific visual images—a day at the beach and a walk in the forest, for example—that were designed to make them relax, and listen carefully to the rhythm of their breathing.

In minutes, Terry was totally relaxed. Focusing on his breath had erased the mind chatter that shadowed his every waking thought and allowed him to concentrate on the visualization. It also meant he was more receptive to the entire process.

"At some point, I was told to send peaceful thoughts to my headache," says Terry. "To see the negative energy present in my head that was creating the aches, then replace it with pure, clean, calm, healing energy." It was like visualizing a dark cloud, then seeing it change in your mind's eye to a cloud full of white radiance.

"It was much more than just positive thinking," says Terry. "I was actively working to release the headache from my mind and body."

The result? As the end of the seminar approached, Terry noticed that a deep calm had engulfed his entire body. "For the first time in years I felt no pain," he says. "The headache was gone."

Terry was stunned.

"Being a skeptic, I was tempted to go back inside my head to find the headache. I wanted to search for it so I could disprove what had happened. But the group leader told me not to because I could easily create another headache in the process.

"I left that seminar with a new sense of power," says Terry. It was to that power he turned when faced with surgery.

FOCUSED ON HEALING

Terry decided to give visualization a try right after his chiropractor had diagnosed the slipped disk. At first, "I was frightened," says Terry. "The pain was so bad I didn't know how I was going to calm my mind long enough to begin the visualization.

"Painkillers were out of the question because I needed a clear head, so I took it minute by minute. I kept telling myself, 'If I can outlast the pain this minute, then I can do it for the next, and the next after that.'"

Terry spent the next forty-eight hours practicing the visualization technique he had learned. First he did breathing exercises to relax and make it easier to concentrate. "I'd start by following my breath for twenty minutes at a time," Terry says. "With my eyes closed, I'd take a deep breath and hold it in for a few seconds, then let it out, and in my mind, I followed my breath as it went in and out of my body. I did it until my mind was completely focused on my breath, and I eventually lost track of whether I was inhaling or exhaling, or where one breath started and the other ended. It worked like a sedative."

Did the pain actually subside?

"I kept looking for the pain to end," says Terry. "Then I realized: By looking for the pain, I was directing energy toward recreating it. So each time my mind took me near the pain, I went back to focusing on my breath. When I was finally able to stay focused on my breath, an incredible calm engulfed my body, and I experienced some relief for the first time in hours.

"It's not that the pain went away," he adds. "But it lessened enough so that I could focus my mind on using the visualization.

"I imagined my spine fusing together, the disks going back into place, me walking and eventually running pain-free. I kept those images in my mind, and every time a negative image popped up, I'd replace it with a positive one. I saw myself going from paralyzed to walking, from pain-filled to pain-free, from stiff to flowing, from unhealthy to healthy."

Within a few days, Terry was well enough to be moved from his bed in Idaho back home to California. He visited several doctors, including an orthopedist who took x rays, noted a defect in how Terry's sacrum was built, and confirmed the slipped disk.

"I used the x rays that were taken as part of my visualization," says Terry. "I had a chiropractor show me what normal and healthy vertebrae, nerves, and disks looked like, then what my damaged disks looked like. Then I closed my eyes and visualized the diseased back as though it were on a large screen. I would visualize it fading into the distance and then a healthy back slowly reappearing and coming closer. I did this for five to ten minutes every day for ten days, then on and off for another thirty days or so.

"Some days the visualization was more like a sense, a knowing. Other days it was in Technicolor, 70 mm, digital Dolby sound."

One month later, to the amazement of his doctors, Terry was up and—if not running, at least hobbling.

"It took a couple of months until everything returned to normal, but eventually, I returned to full body motion," he says. "I continued the visualization at least once a day for several more weeks, and I've used it since to help with everything from sports injuries to toothaches. The more I use this technique, the better and faster results seem to come.

"When I first started doing the relaxation part, for example, it would take me upwards of twenty minutes to complete. I achieve the same results now within a couple of minutes."

A NEW LIFE

Although visualization's primary value to Terry is the way in which it allows him to handle pain and heal his body, it has also affected his life in other positive ways. Most important, perhaps, it has led him to a deeper reflection about the relationship between mind and body, and a deeper respect for both.

"I know this must sound crazy," admits Terry, "but by choosing this alternative technique over surgery or painkillers, I was able to take the time to see what the pain was trying to tell me about the way I had been running my life."

For Terry, this was critical information, having lost both his father and grandfather to heart attacks by their fifty-ninth birthdays.

"My father and his father before him were both successful businessmen," explains Terry. "And I was taught to strive for the American dream—financial success—at any cost.

"But the more I focused on success, the more obsessed I became with succeeding—and it took a toll on my body. I was far more concerned with how far my body could take me before it collapsed than worrying about any future damage I might have been causing it."

For Terry, this accident was an eye-opener, helping him to redefine aspects of his life that, he felt, if left unchanged, would have resulted in major health problems. "I believe," reflects Terry, "one of the primary reasons my back gave out the way it did was because I was living my life fairly rigidly, not listening to my intuitions and needs." Where once Terry was afraid that he'd follow the men in his family down the road to heart attacks and other serious medical conditions, he now feels that with his commitment to a better diet, more relaxed lifestyle, and greater attunement to his body's needs through creative visualization, he can lead a healthy, active life well into old age.

The result? Today, Terry is a different person. The martinis, caffeine, and fast food are a thing of the past, and his pace is far less hectic. That's not to say that Terry is not a busy man. He still runs a number of business ventures—real estate in Oregon, wine in Bulgaria, executive team-building seminars in California—and in his "spare" time, he photographed and wrote a book about the coming down of the Berlin wall. He also leads groups of business executives on wilderness adventures on Idaho's rivers.

If you're lucky enough to find yourself on one of Terry's adventures, don't be surprised if before entering the river he suggests closing your eyes for a creative visualization process prior to donning your life jacket to help make your journey on the rapids the ride of your life.

SPOTLIGHT ON CREATIVE VISUALIZATION

Creative visualization is the way your mind speaks to your body. Visualize a slice of chocolate cake and your salivary glands will pump out the extra enzymes you need to digest it. Visualize your body healing a molecule or two of a virus—as researchers have done in the lab—and your body's immune system will suddenly zip up its production of warrior antibodies to attack the viral invader.

It's a technique that has been used by artists, actors, writers, architects, city planners, mathematicians, musicians, and athletes to create a particular vision within the "mind's eye" that allows them to create a new reality. In the visualization, they can rehearse, plan, or even analyze problems from a new perspective.

World-class athletes are particularly known to use this technique to rehearse every nuance of a performance before they compete. Olympic diver Greg Louganis, track star Jackie Joyner-Kersey, and tennis superstar Martina Navratilova use visualization on a regular basis. So does tennis ace Gabriella Sabatini, who attributes at least one U.S. Open victory to this process: "I pictured winning every point," said Sabatini after beating Steffi Graf. "I visualized winning the whole tournament."

How was this powerful mind/body language discovered? Nobody really knows. But its value has been understood at least from the time that the Roman philosopher Marcus Aurelius said sagely, "Life is what our thoughts make it."

The first attempts to scientifically document that idea seem to have occurred in the 1930s, when researcher Edmund Jacobson found that if you visualize yourself doing some particular action—kicking a ball with your right foot, for example—the muscles that control movement in that area will show increased electrical activity just as if they were actually carrying out the motion.

No one really knew what this information meant, although researchers played around with it for decades. But in 1971, pioneering radiologist and cancer specialist O. Carl Simonton, M.D., decided to see if visualization could help cancer patients increase their chances of survival.

Dr. Simonton first had his patients relax, then instructed them to visualize the cancer in their bodies replaced with healthy and functioning cells.

His earliest work involved using this visualization three times a day with a sixty-one-year-old throat cancer patient whom the medical community had written off. The man was having difficulty breathing and swallowing and was in such a weakened state that no one thought he could endure the aggressive radiation treatments that might help him survive.

Under Dr. Simonton's guidance, the patient began to use visualization. For five to fifteen minutes three times a day, he imagined radiation treatments as energy bullets that were fired at his cells. Healthy cells were to be visualized as being energized by the bullets, while cancer cells were to be visualized as being killed. The visualization was completed with the man imagining the cancer shrinking and his health returning to normal.

The result? The man's health improved just enough so that Dr. Simonton could perform the necessary radiation therapy. Within two months after radiation, the man's cancer went into remission.

Although one successful case history does not prove that any treatment works, this one literally changed the course of science. Millions of dollars of research funds have been allocated to investigate how visualization might work and how it can effectively be used as an adjunct to traditional medical therapies.

So far the technique has been found effective in treating a host of common ailments such as back pain, eyestrain, headaches, skin ailments, irregular menstruation, and sports injuries of all kinds. It is a perfect antidote to stress, which is an underlying factor in many diseases. As with Dr. Simonton's cancer patient, it also seems to be effective in helping people improve the odds of traditional therapies such as surgery. Visualization has not been proven to cure serious diseases such as cancer on its own, however, as some proponents have claimed.

Although visualization is believed to work on a physical level by allowing the mind to program the body's healing mechanisms, experts say that there are psychological benefits to using visualization as well.

That's because the process itself frequently provides valuable insights into emotional problems that may underlie or exacerbate an illness. In fact, trained therapists sometimes encourage patients to use visualization to "talk" with a particular part of their body that is ill or in pain. This actually gives a "voice" to the pain or illness, and, in therapist-directed self-chats, enables the patient to figure out what caused the underlying emotional problem and how it should be handled. Thus the patient's health, as a whole, is enhanced.

A therapist might begin the visualization process by asking you to sit down, close your eyes, take a deep breath, and imagine that you're taking a walk in the forest, watching the ocean at sunset, or lying in a field of lilies. Use all of your senses to visualize the scene: Smell the lilies, hear the sound of the waves, feel the grass under your toes, or taste the salt air as you walk along the beach.

Then once you are completely relaxed, the therapist might suggest, as Dr. Simonton did with his cancer patient, that you think of a particular image and see it working to fix a particular health problem. A cancer patient might visualize his body's natural killer cells attacking a tumor, while someone with back pain might visualize a cleaning crew sponging up all the pain chemicals released by the body and wringing them out in the bladder for disposal out of the body.

You can follow this process on your own, and many people report good results in as little as two ten-minute sessions a day.

A good way to get started is to visit your local bookstore to gather more information on how people use the technique to deal with specific problems. There you'll find a plethora of books, audiotapes, and even videotapes that explain how various practitioners have adapted the technique to meet their own needs. You might also contact your local YMCA or community center to see if introductory classes are scheduled.

Don't be afraid to plunge right in and try the technique yourself. The next time you have a headache, for example, take a moment prior to popping an aspirin to try visualization. Sit down, close your eyes, take a deep breath, and try to imagine what your headache looks like. Is it a bunch of little guys with hammers running rampant through the back of your head? Is it a heavy rock weighing down the spaces behind your eyes? A jackhammer at your temples?

Now try visualizing a superbly healthy, all-powerful hero who rounds up these nasty guys, rolls away that rock, or pulls the plug on the jackhammer. Keep visualizing his efforts for about ten minutes. Don't look at your watch; just estimate the time, then open your eyes.

So where's your headache?

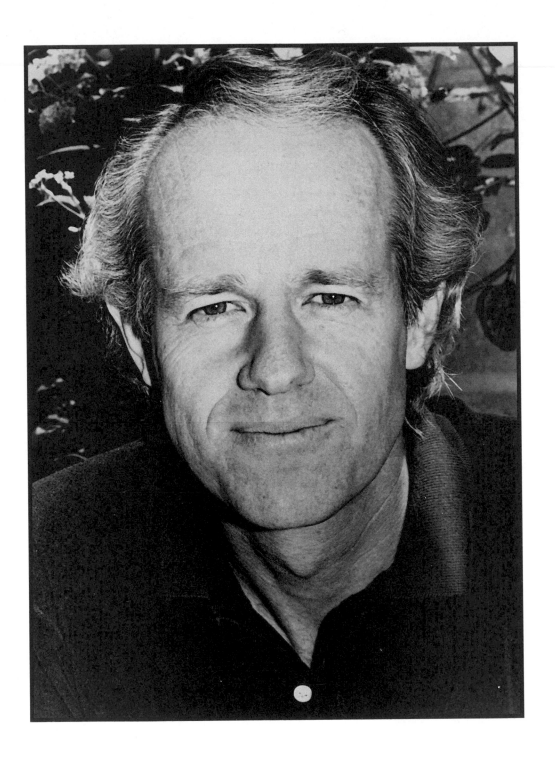

6 ENVIRONMENTAL MEDICINE

BORN
1939, South St. Paul, Minnesota

CAREER HIGHLIGHTS
Co-Chair, Human Rights Watch
Spokesperson, Concern/America

TELEVISION
"M*A*S*H"
"Days of Our Lives"
"The Interns"
"Sex and the Single Parent"
"Prime Suspect"
"Memorial Day"
"Choices of the Heart"
"Private Sessions"
"Hart Attack"

THEATER
Clarence Darrow

"The whole thing has been an extraordinary life-affirming process."

At fifty-six, Mike Farrell is a man who knows about a great many things. He knows how to act, direct, and produce, and how to be a great husband and son. And when it comes to his health, the man who leapt into our hearts as Dr. B. J. Honeycutt, Alan Alda's surgical sidekick on the hit TV series "M*A*S*H," Mike knows one more thing: He doesn't want to follow his father into an early grave.

"My father was a powerful man," explains Mike. "He was a meat-and-potatoes, beer-drinking laborer who worked as a carpenter and prop maker. He was popular and big and strong and healthy, yet when I was ten, as we were driving, he would stop the car and walk over to the side of the road to vomit. He had stomach ulcers. As a result of his illness, I saw him reduced to a victim."

Mike was fifteen when his father's ulcers were surgically removed. Mike recalls: "I vividly remember watching him being wheeled off into the operating room and not knowing if I would ever see him again."

Mike's father survived the surgery, but he died not long after of a heart attack—a devastating event that still deeply affects Mike in more than just the obvious ways.

"Watching my dad's misery and the inability of the medical community to do anything about it was difficult for me," admits Mike. "It just didn't make any sense. Here we are with this extraordinary medical system, only to have it break down."

Fueled by the memory of his father, Mike decided to take control of his own health problems. "For me," recalls Mike, "the turning point came when my prostate became inflamed and I went to a medical specialist for help." The doctor diagnosed Mike's problem as prostatitis, an inflammation of the prostate common in men over the age of fifty.

But this was the second time in six months that Mike's prostate had become inflamed. And if antibiotics didn't zap the underlying infection the first time, Mike figured he'd better find another alternative.

"It's not that I didn't believe in the use of antibiotics," Mike says. "I know that there are times when they're the only viable solution to specific health problems. But I didn't want to be dependent on them. And I believed that there were other solutions that would work just as well without side effects, like robbing my body of valuable bacteria that keep the intestinal tract in good working order.

"If there was an alternative that worked in harmony with my body, I wanted to find it," says the actor.

A SEARCH FOR WHOLENESS

Mike began his search for an alternative health therapy with three goals in mind: One, he wanted to get rid of his prostate problems once and for all; two, he wanted to know more about the connection between his health and the environment, something that was of growing concern; and three, he wanted an alternative that would take into consideration his diet, the environment, and even the people with whom he was interacting.

Eventually Mike's search led him to an alternative health care practitioner who had studied nutrition and herbs. The practitioner told Mike his prostatitis could be treated in a more natural way than using prescription drugs, and the herbs he prescribed seemed to do the trick.

This success piqued Mike's interest in using natural methods to heal. But as his interest evolved, the actor began to realize that many health problems could be prevented if only people would take a closer look at their environment.

One man who helped him realize that was Matt Van Benschoten, a doctor of Oriental medicine whom Mike met in Reseda, California. Dr. Van Benschoten specializes in environmental medicine, a stepchild of the more accepted medical discipline of allergy and immunology. Many of those who practice environmental medicine—some of whom may actually be medical doctors—feel that man-made chemicals in our water, air, and soil kick the immune system into a hyper-responsive state in a largely futile effort to eliminate the chemicals from our bodies. The effort also generates a number of symptoms—fatigue, swelling, inflammation, rashes, itchiness, and headache —that are synonymous with an immune system in overdrive.

Although Mike showed none of these symptoms, Dr. Van Benschoten checked for the health effects of any environmental influences using Omura's test, a test of grip strength between the middle finger and thumb on the patient's right hand. Mike made a circle with his thumb and middle finger while Dr. Van Benschoten sequentially exposed him to open containers of various medications and chemicals; if Mike's fingers became weak, it indicated that he was allergic or sensitive to the substance to which he was being exposed.

Dr. Van Benschoten also checked Mike's acupuncture points—specific points on the body where, according to Chinese belief, the body's "life force" can be redirected—to see if there were any weak areas in his system as a result of environmental factors.

The tests revealed that Mike was healthy. The actor had already made changes to his diet over the years—he ate no meat and drank only bottled water—but with Dr. Van Benschoten's help he was able to define other environmental strategies that would best support his continued good health well into old age.

Each person's prescription for good health varies with individual needs and the environment in which the person exists, according to environmental medicine specialists. By examining the individual in relation to everything he eats, breathes, and touches in his environment, any sensitivities or allergens in the environment that might cause headaches, runny noses, rashes, or even difficulty breathing might be identified and removed—before they cause trouble.

"I began to see Dr. Van Benschoten every two months or so for preventive health care," says Mike. "Each visit I would bring in things [that] he would test to see how they could possibly affect me."

It was on one of these visits that Dr. Van Benschoten discovered some dairy residue and trace antibiotics in Mike's body. The doctor's prescription? A combination of herbs that would eliminate the residue and boost Mike's immune system. Mike was told to give up dairy foods, which Dr. Van Benschoten believed to be the source of the antibiotics.

"The doctor told me how the entire dairy-eating population was being affected by the use of bovine growth hormones. The studies he had read indicated that the widespread use of these hormones was tripling the incidence of udder infections in cattle. The cattle producers' response was to triple the use of animal tetracycline. The doctor was beginning to see a large number of patients who were manifesting signs of animal antibiotics, which he traced back to the dairy products they were eating."

Dr. Van Benschoten explains: "When it comes to dairy, I've come to believe that bovine products are good for bovines and that's it. In the past, my patients could get away with a little dairy here and there, which did clog them up, creating excess mucus, sinus infections, sore throats, and other common ailments. But, with all of the hormones and antibiotics that are now being pumped into bovine, I can no longer recommend it as a part of anyone's diet."

Mike's wife, Shelley Fabares, who stars in the long-running television show "Coach," joined him in his efforts to lead a healthier life and also decided to avoid dairy products. But it wasn't easy, Mike notes with a smile that recalls some of their early struggles.

"You've got to understand, before my wife and I got together twelve years ago, she was a Tootsie Roll–eating, M&M-popping, cigarette-smoking woman," Mike chuckles.

Today, of course, Shelley no longer eats either of those foods, nor does she smoke. Both she and Mike eat lots of fresh fruits and vegetables—generally organically grown—drink bottled water, and have drastically cut back on red meat.

"Not everybody needs to become a vegetarian," says Dr. Van Benschoten. "My wife is a petite, strong woman who does very well eating lots of red meat every day. But even at 6'1", I would be in the hospital if I ate anywhere near the meat she eats. It's a very individual thing that people need to be individually evaluated and tested for.

"If you're going to eat meat and chicken, however, it should be hormone-free, free-range meat and poultry," says Dr. Van Benschoten. These meats are grown differently than most store-bought meats—without growth hormones, antibiotics, and other potentially harmful drugs.

Once Mike and Shelley were comfortable that their diet was free of any potentially unhealthy environmental influences, they turned their attention to their home. Mike put water filters on all the faucets in the house, and they traded in all their toxic household cleaners for environmentally friendly household products.

"I won't use heavy-duty cleaning products for grit and grime," Mike says. "And even when it comes to something like drain cleaning, my weapon of choice is baking soda and vinegar. Together they form an acid that can break through just about anything, and you don't have to inhale any fumes."

On a personal level, "we try not to use aerosols or room fresheners," Mike says. "And my deodorant, shampoos, and toothpaste are always made from natural products that are purchased at a health food store."

Crediting his dedication to alternative health care, Mike's fear that he'd follow the same path as his father to ill health and early death is now a distant memory. "Now," says the healthy actor, "I'm stunned by the fact that I'm fifty-six and feel like I'm twenty."

HELP FOR MOM

Not long after Mike and Shelley had gotten their life on a healthy track, Mike's eighty-eight year-old mom developed severe back pain.

"My mother was in pure agony," Mike recalls. "I took her to an orthopedist, who took x rays. He said my mother had fractured a cervical vertebra. His solution was to prescribe painkillers and sleeping pills, but his treatment soon escalated to a series of medications, one after another. Eventually the doctor decided she needed a back brace and, of course, more painkillers."

The drugs never deadened the pain completely, and Mike began to be concerned about whether the drugs' side effects were worth the relief his mother did get. "My mother became irritable and started experiencing sleep problems," says the actor. She also began to experience headaches, tingling, numbness, and shaking limbs.

Not knowing which symptoms were due to side effects from the drugs and which were caused by pressure on nerves from osteoporosis or the cracked vertebra, the family kept taking Mike's mom to new doctors. The final straw came when Mrs. Farrell was taken to a pain clinic at the recommendation of an internist. The doctors at the clinic tried combinations of drugs and injections until, as Mike put it, "the day that the doctor was lucky I wasn't there to hear his words, 'cause I might have punched him." The doctor threw up his hands and announced, "She's going to have to learn to live with a lot of pain the rest of her life."

At that point, Mike asked her to see Dr. Van Benschoten and she agreed. She'd seen him once before, and he hadn't been able to help. But this was desperate. Everyone else had given up on solving her problem. So she agreed to give him another chance.

Dr. Van Benschoten examined Mike's mom, testing her reactions to hundreds of different common chemicals and asking questions about her diet and environment. "He told us that the problem with my mother was that she had an irritated nerve as a result of pressure from her osteoporosis. Her lungs were also infected," Mike said. The doctor diagnosed her shaking was due to contamination of her water supply with trichloroethylene (TCE), an industrial solvent and degreaser that has contaminated about 3 percent of all groundwater supplies in the United States. Given that she was still drinking tap water, he asked her to bring in a sample; his diagnosis proved to be correct.

Dr. Van Benschoten told Mike's mom to start drinking bottled water. In about six months, she was symptom-free. "Her back pain went away and she looked great," says the actor. "The medical doctors said she would wear a back brace and be on painkillers for the rest of her life. While she still wears the back brace on occasion, she is now drug-free."

Although a young Mike Farrell may not have been able to change his father's destiny, an older Mike clearly changed not only his own path to health but his mother's as well. "Seeing her well was a tremendous relief for all of my family," Mike says. "The whole thing has been an extraordinary life-affirming process."

SPOTLIGHT ON ENVIRONMENTAL MEDICINE

Ever wonder what the pesticides on your lawn are doing to your health as you walk across that lovely expanse of green? Or the fumes from your dry cleaning? How about the constant inhalation of solid room deodorizers?

Scientists suspect that frequent exposure to these substances may not be all that conducive to a healthy existence. So while laboratory scientists are hard at work figuring out exactly how the constant bombardment of man-made chemicals affects the human organism, a new medical specialty has evolved to help people cope with what seems to be a rash of health problems that arise from exposure to the toxic chemicals and cancer-causing agents we commonly toss around our environment.

Called environmental medicine, this specialty demands that people look at the contribution environmental factors play in producing illness. The trailblazer in this area was Theron Randolph, M.D., a medical professor and allergy specialist in the 1940s who first made the connection between the foods we eat and the hives, eczema, fatigue, and headaches that can indicate a sensitivity or allergy to them. In 1962 he wrote the first textbook on the subject, *Human Ecology and the Susceptibility to the Chemical Environment.*

Environmental physicians believe there are any number of both man-made and natural agents that affect our health, including pollens, molds, pesticides, chemicals, foods, food preservatives, petroleum products, and plastics, among others. Although people who work in the manufacturing or application of man-made chemicals may be most severely affected, all of us are exposed to these substances on a regular basis.

Even in our daily environments, environmental physicians find risks of adverse health consequences through the cleaning fluids used to dry-clean our clothing, the bathroom cleaner we use to wash the tub and tiles of built-up grime, the fumes we inhale when filling up our cars at a gas station, the pesticide residue on fruits and vegetables, or even the chemicals used to clean our drinking water. The list of possibly harmful substances is endless.

Everyone is affected to a different degree by these potentially harmful substances. Pollens affect some and not others. Food additives send some running to the bathroom while others stare after them in astonishment. And while some people can wear strong perfumes, scented deodorants, and hair products without so much as a sniffle, other people find themselves sneezing and congested after a single exposure. Some people are so severely affected that they develop a headache and nausea when they simply smell one of these products on another person who happens to be riding in the same elevator. What's more, so many people react to the food additive monosodium glutamate (MSG) that restaurants not using it frequently boast about it on their menus.

Other symptoms include runny nose, clogged nasal and ear passages, blurred vision, itchy skin, diarrhea, chest tightness, shortness of breath, fluid retention, swelling of any number of organs or limbs, poor circulation, muscle spasms, arthritic pain, sleep disorders, asthma, hives, sexual dysfunction—the list goes on and on.

These symptoms can be triggered either by an allergy or a sensitivity to various environmental agents. Generally speaking, a sensitivity is a reaction that everyone will have to a particular substance, although to varying degrees. Everyone will have a reaction when exposed to polyurethane, for example. Depending upon such factors as ventilation, in some people the reaction will be significant enough to notice—a headache, for example—while in others it won't be detectable.

An allergy is different even though it manifests some of the same symptoms. It's an immune system reaction that occurs in only some people, generally those who are genetically predisposed to it. If one person in a family is allergic to tree pollen, for example, there's a good chance that someone else in the family will be as well.

Medical doctors have known about allergies for years and are generally well-prepared to treat their symptoms with an arsenal of medication or immunotherapy—a system of customized shots designed to teach your immune system to stop reacting to an allergen.

But some physicians still reject the idea that the human body can be severely affected by sensitivities; that's where environmental physicians have evolved to fill the gap. Not only can they treat allergies with standard medicines and practice, but they can also assist their patients by helping them sort out what in their environment might be triggering a sensitivity reaction. This is particularly important, say environmental specialists, because continued exposure to agents that cause sensitivity reactions may lead to serious illnesses such as cancer and respiratory failure.

Alternative practitioners of environmental medicine perform tests for sensitivities using muscle testing and checking acupuncture points, as well as checking diet and household environmental contaminants.

The first task at hand for an environmental physician is to figure out, through diagnostic testing, exactly what chemicals or allergies are affecting the person's health. Most allergies can be diagnosed through blood and skin tests, although some physicians prefer to diagnose food allergies through an elimination diet, in which the patient removes the suspected allergen from the diet for a period of two weeks. If allergy symptoms disappear during that time, then reappear when the food is reintroduced, there's a good chance the person is allergic to that particular food.

Environmental physicians generally believe that everything from autism to PMS can benefit from paying attention to what substances in the environment may be involved in causing symptoms. Some of the problems they believe can be alleviated include hyperactivity, seizures, depression, menstrual problems, and prostate problems. They also are investigating the role environmental toxins such as pesticides play in brain disorders that cause memory loss and concentration.

Once diagnosed, most patients will generally be advised to eliminate any agent to which they have allergic or sensitivity reactions. In some instances where avoidance is not possible, physicians will prescribe a variety of antihistamines and/or other medications designed to reduce symptoms. Some doctors also will use food supplements, acupuncture, and herbal remedies that they feel will help.

Alternative practitioners of Oriental medicine, acupuncturists, chiropractors, and homeopaths are often trained in technologies that can help diagnose environmental sensitivities. When calling for an appointment, ask about the practitioner's expertise in this area.

But while you're waiting for an appointment, start keeping a symptom diary. Write down all the things you do each hour during the day. Include all the foods you eat, the chemicals to which you're exposed, and any symptoms that occur. Look around your house and work environment, list the products you use to wash your clothes, your body, and your home. Even the kinds of candles you burn may affect your health. This can greatly assist your doctor in identifying potentially harmful products you may be using.

And to get started on your environmentally healthy lifestyle, you may want to consider eliminating dairy products from your diet and buying organically grown fruits and vegetables. If you do eat pesticide-drenched produce, scrub or peel it to remove as much residue as you can.

Ditch your petroleum-based cleaners and use citrus-based cleaning products instead. Start hanging your just-back-from-the-cleaners clothes outside or in an unused closet until the fumes dissipate. When filling your car with gas, position yourself upwind from the pumps to avoid inhaling gas fumes. If you are having your home painted, plan on being away for the painting and drying period when many harmful toxins linger. Latex paints have less fumes than oil-based paints, and they dry quicker. Make sure those painting your home use floor fans to exhaust fumes—both for your sake and theirs. What kind of pots do you cook in? Aluminum? This, too, could have negative effects on your health.

Finally, the next time ants invade, forget the insecticide.

Use your foot.

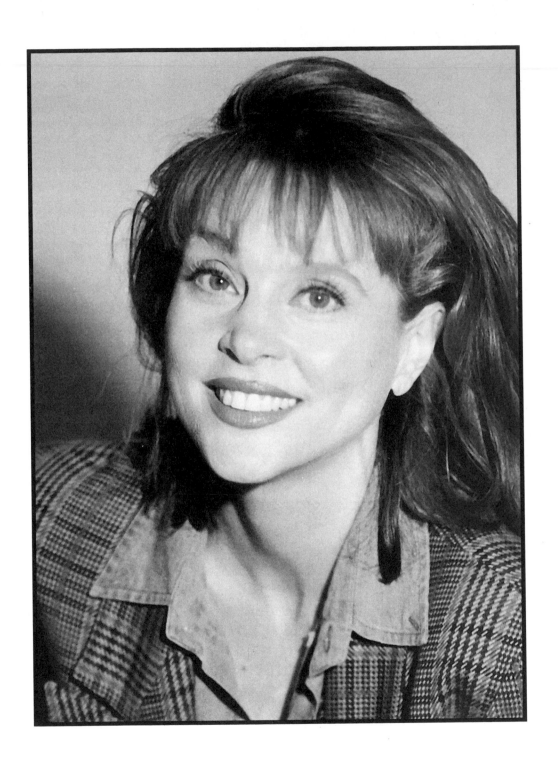

LEIGH TAYLOR-YOUNG
ACTRESS

7 FENG SHUI

BORN
Washington, D.C.

EDUCATION
Northwestern University

PROFESSIONAL AWARDS
Emmy Award,
Best Supporting Actress, 1993:
"Picket Fences"

PROFESSIONAL HIGHLIGHTS
FILM
Jagged Edge
Looker
Soylent Green
*The Gang That Couldn't
Shoot Straight*
The Horsemen
I Love You, Alice B. Toklas

TV SERIES
"Dallas"
"Peyton Place"
"Perry Mason: The Case of the
Sinister Spirit"

THEATER
Sleeping Dogs
Three Bags Full
The Beckett Plays

"I stumbled upon feng shui by chance. I thought, 'This sounds intriguing—I'm going to give it a try.' I especially enjoyed the feng shui money ceremony. But after receiving a surprise check in the mail for $20,000, who wouldn't?"

Leigh Taylor-Young was ready for a change.

The Emmy Award–winning actress—as beautiful as the day she first said hello to television audiences as the breathtaking ingenue of "Peyton Place"—had lost her home, lost her father to cancer, and was in the process of getting a divorce.

Although she had no problem getting a part here and there, when she returned full time to her acting career after a five-year sabbatical to pursue her spiritual development, the chauffeured limousines that studios routinely sent to carry her around town no longer stopped at her curb. Leigh had lost momentum.

"This is an industry that waits for no one," says Leigh. "I had to start from what felt like ground zero, auditioning for parts that in earlier days would have been offered to me outright. And believe me, I was grateful for any work I could get."

Leigh persevered, but it looked like she was running out of luck.

But one day at the gym, Leigh noticed an unusual, eight-sided figure printed on the wall. She studied the figure for a moment, then forgot it as her trainer arrived. But later that day at her acupuncturist, she saw the figure again, this time executed as a framed octagonal mirror hanging in the waiting room. Sitting on a table near the hanging, almost as though it were part of an intentional arrangement, was a book on feng shui, the 2,000-year-old Chinese art form that uses the home and office as a backdrop and the interior layout—furniture, plants, wind chimes, art—to form an environment that will capture *chi*, a kind of life energy.

Leigh was curious. Picking up the book, she leafed through its pages and found that arranging the home or office's contents in accordance with feng shui principles symbolized in an eight-sided figure—called a *bagua* by the Chinese—could reenergize the environment's *chi* and bring luck.

"The more I read about feng shui, the more I liked it," Leigh says. "It was all very intriguing."

MYSTICAL INTERIOR DESIGN

Leigh's acupuncturist referred her to Janet Durovchic, a feng shui expert who had helped arrange the acupuncturist's office in feng shui form.

Janet set up an appointment to look at Leigh's Hollywood apartment, which doubled as both home and office, but asked Leigh to find out something about the apartment's history before the two met.

What Leigh found out shocked her. "Since moving into my apartment, I had had difficulty sleeping at night," says Leigh. "It took a bit of work, but I found that the man who lived here before me had burned himself to death in the bedroom."

When Janet arrived, Leigh told her the news. Janet was disturbed. The Chinese believe that when you move into a new environment, you can be influenced by both the good and bad experiences, the *chi*, that linger from previous tenants. In Leigh's case, the pain and violence of the previous tenant's death affected both the environment and Leigh.

Concerned about the possibility, Janet performed a feng shui ceremony called a house blessing that tradition taught would clear out any old energies that might have lingered.

Did it work? "I can truly say that for the first time since moving into my apartment, I experienced a real calm in my bedroom after Janet completed her house blessing," says Leigh.

Janet also felt the change. She proceeded to analyze the apartment's *chi* from a feng shui perspective.

Using the eight-sided *bagua* almost as a topographical map, Janet checked to see that each of the eight "power centers" on the *bagua* that symbolized wealth, helpful people, marriage and relationships, children, reputation, career, knowledge, and family were present—and in the same configuration—in the apartment. [See illustration, page 79.]

In feng shui tradition, the absence of any one of these eight centers indicates that it could be absent from your life. Using the entrance to your home as an orientation point, the feng shui expert will check to see all centers are represented.

Janet had seen several cases where clients with a missing "relationship" center complained to her of "something" missing in their marriage. "In the worst possible scenario, the couple will divorce," says Janet. "At best, they may cohabit, but find the relationship leaves a lot to be desired."

Equally disturbing is a missing "money" corner or a home where the money center falls in the bathroom. Inhabitants of this type of home often find money hard to hold on to. It may flow in and out of their lives—just like water in and out of the bathroom. One easy change that might help this situation is to place a plant on the toilet tank.

In Leigh's case, Janet discovered that the "helpful people" area was missing. And that, Leigh realized, symbolized certain aspects of her life, especially her career.

"It seemed that for as long as I could remember, I felt like I had been on my own, without much support," Leigh says.

It was a tough road. When she decided to resume her career, even her reputation for talent and hard work was not enough to get her steady employment. She got a few jobs here and there, mostly in television, but nobody really took a deep enough interest in her to give her career a boost.

"Even after my work on the hit series "Dallas" and feature films like *Jagged Edge*, I was still struggling to keep the momentum going," says Leigh.

A NEW BEGINNING

"When the concept of 'helpful people' was introduced, I was ready to embrace it fully," says Leigh. "Reflecting on how I had been doing my career up until that point, I had always assumed being an actress meant having to do it on your own, but then I thought for the first time in a long while, 'Maybe things could be easier, less of a struggle.'

"Janet had me rearrange some of my furniture, including a TV, and add plants and crystals to the [helpful people area] of the apartment," says Leigh. "I also had to regroup a seating arrangement."

All the changes—or "reinforcements," as feng shui advocates refer to them—were designed to invite people who could be benefactors or helpful in some way into Leigh's apartment and into her life. Crystals created a warm and inviting interior as they expanded the capacity for helpful benefactors to come forward. What's more, the television stimulated the area with its electricity, while plants added life by attracting an extra measure of *chi*.

Although more willing to believe that hard work would eventually energize her career, Leigh began to see that making the physical changes Janet suggested would help her to make the inner emotional changes that would enable her to hopefully create more vital connections with some key people who could support her life and career.

"As I made each change in my apartment, inwardly I invited in helpful people," says Leigh. "I used it as a metaphor for my life. I began to make more room inside of me for friends, family, and business associates."

Excited by what she was learning, Leigh was open to other suggestions Janet made about arranging her environment.

Knowing that Leigh really wanted more out of her career, Janet had Leigh create a career power position in her apartment. This involved moving Leigh's desk into a corner of her living room, the career power center in her apartment. "Not everyone would have agreed to place their desk in the living room," says Janet, "but for Leigh this was a real statement of what was important to her."

In addition to making sure that each of the power centers was symbolized in one way or another, Janet also checked the apartment to make sure that the interior layout balanced the male and female energies that make up *chi*, one of the feng shui principles.

It wasn't. The female energy, which had probably been stimulated by Leigh's longtime devotion to spiritual studies, was stronger than the male energy Janet found in the apartment. The male energy, associated with expansion and action, would need to be enhanced.

Janet told Leigh to add a light to the balcony outside of her office so that it would shine on the male portion of her apartment. In feng shui, light is a symbol of strength. By adding light to the masculine part of the house, Leigh was able to give added weight to the masculine side. The result was to balance the apartment between male and female energies.

RICH RESULTS

Since Leigh was also interested in rebuilding her finances as well as her career, Janet suggested Leigh perform a "money ceremony" to help her accumulate wealth.

The main purpose of the ceremony is to remove any obstacles to wealth and prosperity, Janet explained. While we might genuinely desire financial abundance, early childhood patterns, lifetime spending habits, bad luck, and even issues of personal worth can become obstacles to our goal.

The ceremony involves collecting coins of certain denominations and amounts over a twenty-seven-day period and placing them in a bank dedicated to prosperity. At the same time, the person performs ancient prayers and visualizations. Included in the visualization might even be to imagine bank accounts overflowing with large cash deposits.

Although collecting coins, praying, and visualizing are a relatively simple way to focus the individual's attention on a particular goal, some people do find it difficult—mostly because if you forget to perform the ceremony on even one of the twenty-seven days, you have to start all over again from day one.

"It took me a number of restarts, but I finally made it through the twenty-seven days," Leigh says with a laugh.

But the payoff was worth it. "I went to my mailbox a month after I finished the ceremony to find a check in the amount of $20,000," says Leigh. "The money came as a total surprise. It was a royalty check for a show I'd done years earlier, and the money had been accruing."

Leigh also began to feel that her luck had changed in other areas of her life as well. She found "helpful people" in a new management and public relations team she hired, and she was nominated for an Emmy for her role as the mayor in "Picket Fences"—a part she'd landed just before she saw the *bagua* in her acupuncturist's office.

But Leigh doesn't feel that her luck changed just because she rearranged her apartment. "If I had thought that by simply moving my desk, everything in my life would change, I would never have tried feng shui," says Leigh. "Instant cures are about as useful as instant fame." They have a very short life.

Instead, says Leigh, she used feng shui as a metaphor, and as she changed her exterior environment, she also changed the environment within.

"I opened both inwardly and outwardly in a much greater way, drawing people forward to assist me," says Leigh. "Before people would tend to look at me and say, 'She has it all so we don't need to help her.' But after the feng shui, something shifted."

Leigh had created a team of helpful benefactors.

Even old friends sensed the difference and renewed their efforts to help the "new" Leigh. "It was a dear friend who first encouraged me to go after an

Emmy for my work on 'Picket Fences,'" says Leigh. "I hadn't thought much about it as a life goal, but it was through his encouragement that I decided to get behind my producer's Emmy campaign and support it in any way I could."

The result?

Leigh Taylor-Young won the 1993 Emmy for Best Supporting Actress.

SPOTLIGHT ON FENG SHUI

If you think feng shui is only for the rich and famous, think again! While American business executives may not be touting the benefits of a good feng shui session at their board of directors' meetings, many have been secretly pumping this ancient practice into their ventures.

The Dallas–Fort Worth Airport, not content to let its success rest upon its centralized location, employed not one but three feng shui experts to guarantee its continued good fortune.

Creative Artists Agency, a powerful Hollywood talent firm that manages the careers of Tom Cruise, Meryl Streep, Kevin Costner, and Barbra Streisand, employed a feng shui expert to ensure the success of the company's new headquarters.

What's more, when proper placement of an entrance or cash register might mean the difference between no room at the inn and a "vacancy" sign, even Hong Kong's pricey Peninsula hotel employs a feng shui expert.

Feng shui is a 3,000-year-old Chinese form of interior design and exterior placement that is based upon principles first described in the *Li Shu*, a sacred book that establishes the basic tenets of Chinese religious belief.

Literally translated as "wind" and "water," feng shui is designed to create an interior landscape that liberates the environment's *chi* to move as freely as the wind and water of its name, thus bringing the occupant good "luck."

Today feng shui combines that initial theology with 2,000 years of folklore and oral history. Every person who practices or teaches feng shui adds his or her own particular mythology to the mix, but in each instance the intent is to manipulate the outer environment in order to focus our own inner resources, attract support, and achieve our goals.

Feng shui teaches that each room is divided into eight power centers that symbolize wealth, helpful people, marriage, children, reputation, career, knowledge, and family. Objects such as furniture, art, or plants (real or artificial but never dried) are arranged to harmonize the flow of *chi* throughout the home. Prayers and visualizations reinforce the process.

An individual's goal—bearing a child, having money, getting a career boost—will be tied together with one or another of the power centers with related prayers and visualizations designed to focus attention and energy on the achievement of that particular goal.

If a couple is having difficulty conceiving, for example, a feng shui expert will rearrange those parts of their home that correspond to "children" and "family." The expert may suggest the couple hang a crystal attached to a red cord near the location designated as the children's area. The crystal is used to attract *chi* and stimulate its movement throughout the area. The red cord is also used to stimulate *chi*—red is considered a powerful and lucky color in the Chinese culture.

A feng shui expert might also hang a mirror in the family power center. A mirror would serve to double the amount of *chi*, just as it doubles the image of an individual looking into a mirror. In this case, doubling the amount of *chi* in the family segment could remove obstacles that inhibit smooth family interactions.

With prayers and visualizations added to the modified interior, the individual who lived in the home would have created the best possible environment in which to conceive.

How can you get started with feng shui? Rededicate yourself to your own good fortune and try the following:

Take a good look around your living space. Do you feel good about your furnishings, or cringe every time you look at Grandma's old sofa that was too good an offer to refuse?

Get rid of anything that irritates you. Walk through each room, making notes on what you would like to see replaced. If your bed squeaks whenever you get in, and this irritates you, fix it or replace it.

Keep your rooms orderly. A mess does not contribute to a calm, harmonious atmosphere.

Apply the *bagua's* shape over a room in your own home. Augment the areas you would like enhanced in your life with livelier light-increasing objects. While the study and practice of feng shui can be extremely complex and should be performed by an expert, a few simple changes can make a difference. Add the energy of light to dark areas using lead-crystal spheres, mirrors, or electric lights. The addition of healthy plants to dead corners, sharply angled spaces, or in front of windows can be beneficial. If you enter your home only to face a wall, place a mirror there to open up the area for additional good luck.

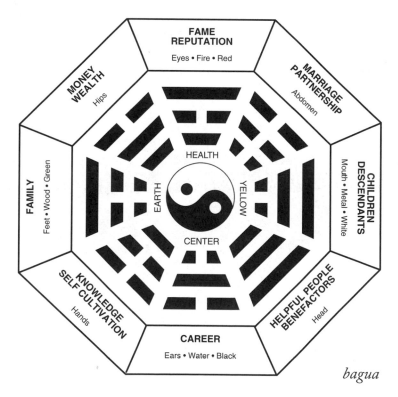

bagua

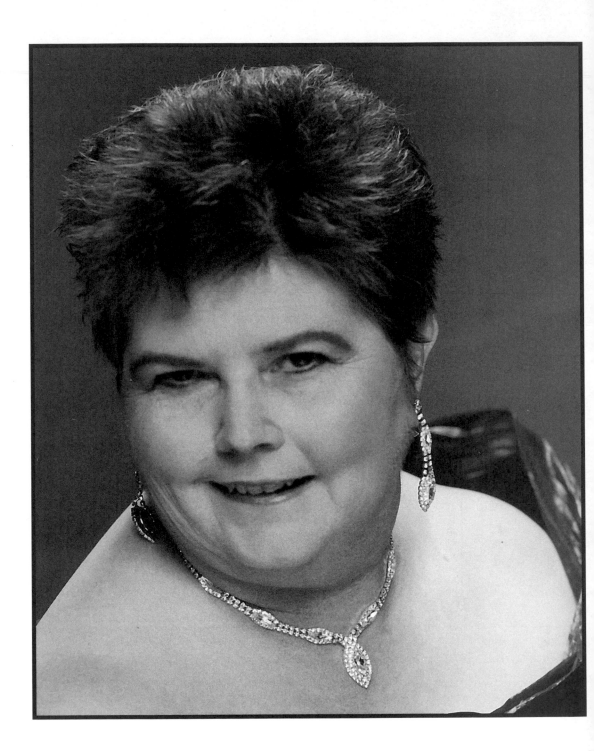

PHYLLIS BIRD
DISNEY ANIMATOR

BORN
1945, Glendale, California

EDUCATION
A.A., Glendale College
Los Angeles Trade Technical

PROFESSIONAL AWARDS
Golden Globe, 1982–83:
Ziggy's Gift

CAREER HIGHLIGHTS
The Black Cauldron
The Little Mermaid
Tummy Trouble for Roger Rabbit
The Great Mouse Detective
Ziggy's Christmas Special
Pocahontas

8 HOMEOPATHY

"Dreams really do come true."

Everyone knows what it's like to have a dream. But Phyllis Bird nearly lost hers to a health problem that threatened to shut down her career.

Phyllis Bird—or "Birdie," as she is affectionately known to friends and fellow animators—is one of those lucky people who had a dream. "From the day my dad gave me a book on how to draw cartoons, I knew what I wanted to do with my life," says Birdie. "I wanted to be an animator, and I wanted to work for Walt Disney, the king of animation."

Who could blame her? After all, how many people get to say that they work on Dopey Drive, receive their job training at Disney University, and never know when Minnie Mouse will sit down next to them at lunch?

Although Birdie is clearly one of those very special people who get to live out their dreams, it took a lot more than wishing upon a star for this particular dream to come true. It took years of hard work and persistence, plus a long search for a real-life fairy godmother—a godmother who would be willing to introduce Birdie to the people who could give her a break. It also took a Cherokee health practitioner to help her keep what she'd won.

Birdie's fairy godmother was an animator in southern California who offered Birdie the chance to assist her on nights and weekends. Knowing it was the first step on the road to realizing her dream, Birdie jumped at the opportunity.

Not that her day job didn't have its share of excitement. "The photo lab where I worked had me doing highly secret government work," says Birdie. "When the film came in to be developed from the Apollo 11 space shuttle, I was the one who got to work on it."

But no matter how much she enjoyed her lab work, Birdie longed to be in animation, to paint life into still-life images and create visual moving masterpieces.

So each day Birdie would hurry from her job at the lab over to her "god-mother's" studio. Then, one special day, she was introduced to the supervisor of paint and ink at Ruby Spears, one of the premier cartoon animation studios in the world.

Once the Ruby Spears people saw what she could do, Birdie's career took off. She had all the work she could handle. But she never lost sight of her dream to work for Disney. So every few years, undaunted by the odds, Birdie would knock on Disney's door and ask for a job.

In 1980, Disney offered Birdie the magic carpet ride of which she had dreamed. The studio was busily preparing a feature animation film, *The Black Cauldron*, and needed additional painters. "The film was very demanding," Birdie says. "I walked in the door and started working seven days a week, eleven hours a day, for eight months straight."

But there were no complaints from Birdie. She was finally working for Walt Disney.

A DISASTER AT DISNEY

Birdie danced on the pinnacle of happiness for nearly five months. Then disaster struck. A skin condition she had ignored for years began to threaten her new job.

"The problem began in my late teens, when I first began working in photography," recalls Birdie. "My hands always seemed to be chapped. Everyone thought it was because I worked with photo and retouch chemicals. But sometimes the part that was chapped would crack open, and I would have gashes in my hands. Doctors said it was just chapping, so I used lotions and tried not to pay too much attention to it."

Over the years the condition worsened. By the time it flared up at Disney, Birdie's hands were a mess. "My hands looked disgusting, so I would wear thin white gloves or wrap them with bandages to hide the lesions. Many times I would go into work and everything would be fine. Then two hours later, the cuts would open up, and my hands would start to ache. It was really awful."

Friends and co-workers were generally sympathetic. "All of us working with paints were used to having dry, chapped hands, so everybody would suggest a favorite lotion," Birdie says. "But the lotions didn't help. And one day, my hands got so bad that a co-worker complained that she was afraid she was going to catch something from me. I was sent home, even though I knew the only person who had a chance of becoming infected was me—the one with the open wounds."

The company suggested that Birdie see a dermatologist. His diagnosis: chronic eczema.

"The dermatologist told me that genetics and stress, along with the chemicals and paints I was working with, could bring it on," Birdie says.

His solution? "Cortisone cream applied topically, along with a huge cortisone shot in my rump."

The treatment worked, but only temporarily. Less than nine months later, Birdie was back in the doctor's office with the same problem. The effects of her second shot were even briefer than the first, and within months,

Birdie's condition returned. At this point, Birdie's doctor gave her one last piece of advice: "If you want to stop the skin condition, quit animation, photo labs, and painting."

Birdie quit animation? Never!

"Can you imagine how I felt?" asks a horrified Birdie. "Being an artist is my whole life. And here he was telling me to give it up. There is no way on God's earth I could stop working with color and art materials."

A REAL SOLUTION

Discouraged by the failure of traditional doctors to treat her hands, Birdie resigned herself to living with the problem. Then, she had a car accident that would change her life.

"I was working on *The Little Mermaid* when I got into a car accident," explains Birdie. "I went to a chiropractor who helped me get my body back into alignment and quickly got me back on my feet." At this point in her career, staying on her feet—and at her art table—was particularly important.

The year was 1990, and the animation industry was about to undergo a revolution: All the animation art that was drawn and painted on paper and cells would be drawn and painted on a computer screen—and Birdie didn't have a clue about how to use computers.

The Little Mermaid would be the last film for which Disney would employ hand painters and inkers, Birdie says. "The art form I had come to know and love would become a thing of the past."

Birdie was concerned that she, too, would become a thing of the past. But after a brief layoff, Disney called her back, trained her on a computer, and put her career back on track.

"I was working on a film called *The Rescuers Down Under* when my back began to give me some trouble again," Birdie says. "So, remembering the success I had had with chiropractic treatment, I decided I would give it another try."

But the chiropractor Birdie visited this time also happened to have an interest in homeopathy—a system that treats a health problem with a highly diluted solution of a substance that causes similar symptoms. This chiropractor thought he could fix not only Birdie's back but her hands as well.

He began by experimenting with different homeopathic remedies. "The first remedy he gave me really didn't work," Birdie says. "He told me that I shouldn't necessarily expect instant relief and that sometimes with chronic problems such as the one I had, it could take some time.

"I took this remedy for some time, and while toward the end I found some relief, it never really gave me the relief I was hoping for. He told me that it may not have been quite the right medicine, so he tried others. I kept waiting for things to get better but they never did. Yet I instinctively felt that with all I had read and heard about homeopathy, there should be a remedy that would work for me. So I kept on trying."

During this time, Birdie was commuting between her work in California and a home she had purchased over the border in Arizona. It was there that a friend referred her to a highly experienced homeopath, Eileen Nauman, HMD, who had been practicing homeopathy for twenty-five years.

"When I first went to see her, my hands weren't as bad as they were during *The Black Cauldron*, but they were still a mess," says Birdie. "We spent about two hours together. She took my full medical history and asked question after question about my life. She seemed to be looking for a bigger picture than just the chemicals around my work environment, and she seemed to be searching for something."

Nauman was. "I was trained to look at a person as a whole, and not just focus on specific symptoms," the homeopath explains. Homeopaths are taught that illnesses are simply a collection of symptoms, and that a variety of factors—both emotional and physical—must be taken into consideration when treating a patient. "Birdie had ailments other than her hands, including digestive problems that rivaled her skin condition," says Nauman. "In addition to the stress of her job, she was just getting over the death of a beloved animal. This, combined with years of being painfully shy, was affecting her emotional state. All of this was affecting her ability to stay healthy. It was only by asking her questions and listening to what was going on in her life, as well as examining her hands, that I was able to treat her."

But by the time Nauman saw Birdie's hands, they looked like raw hamburger, says the homeopath. They were red and slightly swollen with flaps of skin hanging here and there. They also had deep, knifelike cuts that never seemed to quit bleeding. And whenever Birdie got overheated, her hands would get itchy as well.

Birdie decided she wanted to ask Nauman to try to deal with her emotional and digestive problems first. So Nauman first prescribed Aethusa, also known as fool's parsley, to help improve Birdie's state of mind and soothe her stomach.

For three months, Birdie remained on Aethusa and made good progress, according to the homeopath. "Even her shyness seemed to be subsiding," says Nauman. She did not take any other remedy, even for her hands, because to do so might interfere with the Aethusa.

But once Birdie's digestive problems were solved, Nauman turned her attention to Birdie's hands. "I prescribed *Graphites* 12x, a remedy made from carbon, which she was to take three times a day," Nauman says. "Then I told her to call me seven days later and report in."

Birdie followed Nauman's advice. "I took the *Graphites*, which looked like tiny white sugar pills. I put them under my tongue to dissolve for about thirty seconds.

"My homeopath warned me not to touch them with my hands in case my hands had something on them. I had to shake the pills into the bottle cap and take them from there directly into my mouth. I was also told not to eat mints or drink coffee while I was on the remedy because they would interfere with the *Graphites*."

A week later, an ecstatic Birdie called Nauman and reported that 80 percent of her symptoms had disappeared, almost ten years since her hands had begun to interfere with her life.

Knowing they were on the right track, the homeopath continued to prescribe the *Graphites* but increased the potency. Three weeks later, Birdie phoned the doctor again to report her progress. "She told me her hands were completely healed for the first time in her life," says Nauman with obvious satisfaction. "No longer was she bleeding all over the office paper or on her clothes; her hands were soft, had elasticity, and her nails no longer cracked."

A year later, Birdie feels she's been cured. "Every now and then I have minor outbreaks," she admits. "But I simply call my homeopath and she sends me the proper dilution of *Graphites*."

Sound like a dream? The next time you see a Walt Disney film with animation, instead of walking out on the seemingly endless roll of credits that accompany every film, you might want to stick around to see Phyllis Bird's name—if only to remind yourself that dreams really do come true.

SPOTLIGHT ON HOMEOPATHY

Can brushing a poison ivy leaf against your cheek cure a poison ivy rash on your arm? This is the principle behind homeopathy, a form of therapy that is hotly debated among health professionals.

Homeopathy is based on the theory that a disease can be cured with minute amounts of a substance that causes similar symptoms. Since it was first proposed by the German physician Samuel Hahnemann in the late 1800s, it has been attacked and vilified by scientists and defended by its practitioners and patients with equal passion.

The word *homeopathy* combines two Greek words: *homoios* for "like" and *pathos* for "disease," which together describe homeopathy's philosophy that "like cures like." In homeopathy, for example, a person who suffers from hay fever would not be given a medication to suppress a stuffy nose and swollen, itchy eyes. Instead, they would be given a highly diluted solution of a substance that causes similar symptoms. This, homeopaths believe, would stimulate the body's own powers of natural healing.

The only problem is that nobody—not even a homeopath—can explain how homeopathy works. Traditional scientists claim that what works is the placebo effect—the mind's magnificent ability to heal the body roughly one-third of the time no matter what else is done to heal it. Homeopaths refute this argument by citing the multitude of people who say that it works, as well as clinical trials with higher rates of success.

For decades now, Americans traveling through Europe have heard these testimonials. In France and Great Britain, 30 to 40 percent of all prescriptions are written for homeopathic remedies, many of which are available for well under $10.

In France, where pharmacies routinely carry homeopathic remedies, homeopathic cold and flu remedies actually outsell such traditional medicines as decongestant cold capsules. And in Great Britain, even the royal family uses homeopathy.

Homeopathic remedies start out as a solution of a particular substance dissolved in grain alcohol. This "mother tincture" is then diluted over and over again by homeopathic pharmacists. Using one of the formulas these pharmacists employ, for example, one part of the mother tincture is diluted in ninety-nine parts of alcohol. Then one part of this second mixture is again diluted with another ninety-nine parts of alcohol; one part of this third mixture is again diluted with another ninety-nine parts of alcohol. Depending on the mixture, the dilution process can continue another 100,000 times. Depending on whether the mixture has been diluted with ninety-nine parts of alcohol, or nine parts, the mixture is labeled either C or X.

By the time a C mixture has been diluted twelve times or an X mixture has been diluted twenty-four times, the basic rules of chemistry suggest that there's not a single molecule of the original substance left in the solution. But that doesn't bother homeopaths. They believe that the greater the dilution, the more potent the solution. Apparently, shaking the solution between each dilution helps the alcohol "remember" the active ingredient.

Homeopathic remedies are generally processed into tablets and liquids to take orally or gels and tinctures to apply topically.

Homeopaths claim that their remedies can help almost every disease or condition known to humankind. It is a matter of finding the right remedy in the right dosage. And patients say that these remedies are particularly effective in the prevention and treatment of cold, flu, and allergy symptoms, for headaches, menstrual cramps, muscle soreness, dental pain, motion sickness, skin outbreaks, and even emotional ailments such as depression, grief, anxiety, and panic attacks.

Many of the remedies are available in health food stores, but they are also available from the homeopaths who prescribe them.

Homeopaths are frequently health-care professionals—chiropractors, osteopaths, physical therapists, and even medical doctors—who are licensed in their own medical specialty. They then receive additional training in homeopathy. Homeopaths who pass a comprehensive test administered by the American Institute of Homeopathy are permitted to use the initials DMH (doctor of medical homeopathy) or DIMH (diplomate of medical homeopathy) after their names.

Homeopathic practitioners will generally begin treatment with a two-hour consultation that covers not only an assessment of the individual's current health problem, but also a comprehensive evaluation of their emotional and physical state as well. Practitioners then choose the remedy that they feel is most likely to restore the individual to health. Although the initial workup is expensive—between $150 and $500—subsequent visits generally cost $50 to $75. And the remedies are relatively inexpensive.

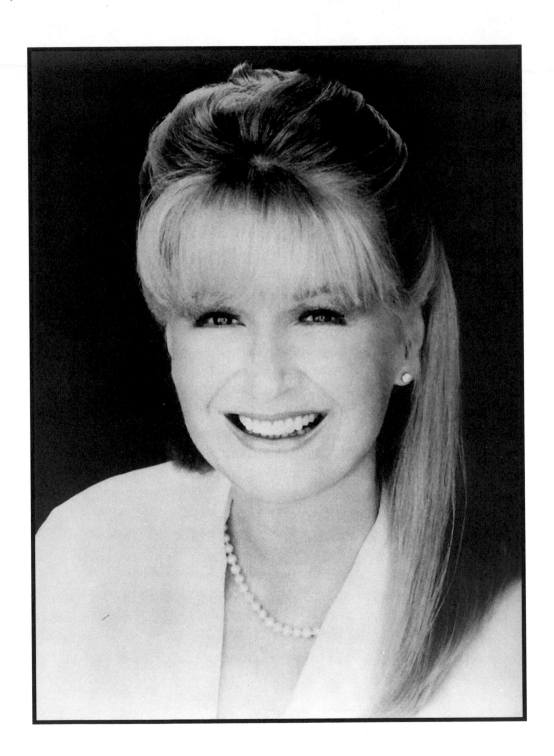

9 JUICING

BORN
1943, Meridian, Mississippi

PROFESSIONAL AWARDS
Three Oscar nominations:
Rambling Rose, Wild at Heart,
Alice Doesn't Live Here Anymore
British Academy Award

CAREER HIGHLIGHTS
FILM
The Cemetery Club
Fatherhood
Christmas Vacation
All Night Long
Chinatown
Wild Angels

THEATER
Hamlet
Noisy Passengers
The Fantastics
Orpheus Descending

TELEVISION
"Alice"
"Thaddeus Rose and Eddie"

"I had become allergic to the theaters in which I was performing. By the end of six weeks on juices, I was totally cured."

AN ALLERGY IN THE THEATER

Diane Ladd may have been named "one of the top ten actors in the world" by *Time,* but given the amount of time she's spent studying nutrition and learning how to maintain a healthy lifestyle with juicing, it's just as easy to imagine her becoming a doctor.

Rose Diane Lanier's acting career was launched when she made her New York stage debut in the production of her cousin Tennessee Williams's *Orpheus Descending.* But it almost crash-landed several years later when she developed an allergy to dust in the theater.

Diane had just divorced actor Bruce Dern, the Broadway play in which she was appearing closed, and she was struggling to raise their daughter, Laura, on her own.

Divorce, lack of work, and single motherhood all took their toll on Diane. It seemed too much for her to handle, and her body began to rebel. "I was stressed out and overloaded," says Diane. "All of a sudden I was allergic to everything. I had difficulty breathing; I felt it in my lungs, and began to talk with an asthmatic wheeze.

"I became allergic to the theaters in which I was rehearsing and performing. Backstage is usually so full of mold that we end up breathing it in."

Then came ragweed and pollen season, and Diane's problems got worse. Her eyes became swollen and teary. She felt awful, and new allergies kept popping up. "I became allergic to my horsehair mattress, my feather pillows, and [my] down comforter," says Diane. "I was also affected by the dust, which was just about everywhere. And, to top it off, I couldn't tolerate being around animals."

Diane's common sense directed her to replace her mattress, pillows, and bedding. But when it came to pets, this daughter of a country vet had a much harder challenge.

"I had just given Laura a sheltie puppy," Diane recalls. "We had it for about three months but I became so allergic to it, I had to give it away."

No matter how heartbreaking an act that was, there was one thing left causing her to suffer that Diane couldn't simply replace or give away: the theaters across the country in which she performed for a living.

Fortunately for Diane, she had inherited a large amount of gumption from her great-grandmother. The doctor, Aunt Prudy, as everyone called her, had studied herbology and the healing arts with the Cherokees.

"Nobody could ever forget the snowy blizzard when she was called out to deliver a baby," recalls Diane. "She got on her horse and got thrown. Even though she broke her leg, she got back up on the horse, rode to where she was needed, delivered that baby, and then went and got her leg set. My great-grandmother was my inspiration," an inspiration that Diane would turn to many times in the coming years.

Diane turned to an allergist.

He gave her a number of "scratch tests," in which minute amounts of potential allergens are injected under the first layer of skin. Then, after waiting fifteen to twenty minutes, red bumps appeared at the test sites of those substances to which Diane was allergic.

"I reacted so strongly to one of the tests that they had to give me something to stop my heart from pounding," Diane says. Diane was experiencing an anaphylactic reaction, which can occur in extremely sensitive people with testing of this kind.

"The tests confirmed that I was allergic to animal dander, ragweed, pollen, dust, and the staph mold that was floating around the theaters. The only problem was the staph in New York theaters was different from the staph in Washington and the staph in Los Angeles."

Diane began a weekly program of allergy shots.

"The shots were effective in stopping most of my symptoms, but I wanted to be cured, not just desensitized," Diane says. "Besides, if you're allergic to animals, you still can't live with puppies. And while the shots prevented most of my discomfort, once I got around things I was allergic to, I still found I reacted."

Nevertheless, Diane continued with the shots until the start of pollen season. "When the ragweed and other pollens came out, my face and body became swollen with excess fluid even though I had been taking weekly shots," the actor says. "Combined with the emotional stress I was under, the allergies made me look like an alcoholic. And I don't even drink!"

Unfortunately, by interfering with Diane's looks, allergies were now interfering with her livelihood.

"I had a film interview, and I knew I couldn't go there with my face all puffy and my body blown up from the fluid I was retaining. It was so bad that I finally went to a doctor. He gave me a diuretic shot to clear the fluid out of my tissue."

It had been nearly eight months since Diane first began the allergy shots when her good friend, Virginia Capers, Tony Award–winning star of the Broadway production *Raisin*, approached her. She had been watching Diane suffer through the allergies.

"Virginia came up to me and handed me a book," Diane recalls. "She said, 'Read this, Diane Ladd.'"

It was a book on the therapeutic effects of juicing.

"I started reading. The book talked about how juicing could be used to cure allergies. So I went out and bought myself some fruits and vegetables, an electric juicer, and began to cure myself.

"Juicing made sense. The book talked about how when your body gets in trouble, the way mine had, you need a lot of vitamins and minerals. And when your body's stressed, or diseased, sometimes there is difficulty in assimilating the supplements. Taking them in liquid form, through juicing, allows the body to digest them much easier," Diane says.

Diane bought a number of books on juicing that offered recipes and juicing regimens for everything from a five-day juice fast to a midday pick-me-up. The books listed exactly what each fruit and vegetable is good for and in what quantities and combinations. It also discussed which ailments are best treated by which juices and how best to prepare them. And fortunately for Diane, they offered a number of recipes for dealing with all kinds of allergies.

"I didn't go on a complete juice fast, but instead decided to supplement my diet with juice," Diane says. "I made and drank four glasses of juice a day out of fresh fruits and vegetables. I also stayed away from the foods I was allergic to." Blood tests by her doctor had revealed that Diane was allergic to corn and mushrooms.

Diane also used colonics, but "mostly I used common sense," says the actress. "I read about what each of the juices was supposed to do—how carrot juice was a good source of beta-carotene; spinach; of B_6; parsley, of bioflavinoids; and how all three were good sources of vitamin A.

"I began to make up drinks juicing fresh bunches of carrots, spinach, cucumber, celery, and parsley, then mixing them together in my juicer." If the produce has a skin, like an orange, you have to peel the fruit first, she adds. The juicer then separates the juice from the pulp.

Within two weeks of beginning her juicing regimen, Diane's allergies began to subside, and she was breathing more easily. "By the end of six weeks on juices, I was totally cured," says the actress. "I gave up the shots and haven't had one since."

It wasn't long before a down comforter found its way back to Diane's bed and Laura's puppy back into the Ladd home. "I was no longer allergic to the puppy," says a gleeful Diane. "That dog ended up living with us until it died eight years later!"

Diane began to study nutrition. She shared the success she had with juicing with her doctors.

"I went back to those doctors and told them what had happened and how my body had been in need of vitamins and nutrients. They said, 'If you eat good meals and have a balanced diet, you don't need to supplement your diet.' But I knew that hadn't been true for me. Sometimes you just have to listen to your own wisdom when it comes to your health."

Now whenever Diane finds herself under a great deal of stress, she knows that it's time to fill up with juices. "I know with all the pressures of the business I'm in, had I not learned the importance of nutrition, I probably wouldn't be around today," says the actress. In fact, today she is a nutrition counselor. And fortunately for the rest of us, Diane has decided to share her knowledge in an upcoming book that contains some of the juicing recipes she developed.

The book also contains Diane's suggestions for using juicing to stay healthy and fight the effects of stress—advice which Diane put to good use when she recently made her directorial debut on the film *Mrs. Munck*. Her co-star that she directed? Ex-husband Bruce Dern.

SPOTLIGHT ON JUICING

Juicers—as people who pulp and squeeze their way through life are playfully called by fellow advocates—are folks who believe in the healing power of natural, unprocessed, unpreserved juice to provide greater health, increased vitality, and radiant beauty.

From the American Medical Association to the American Holistic Health Association, the one thing upon which these diverse experts agree is that eating a balanced diet is the best way to maintain a healthy body, keep your immune system on its toes, provide energy, and prevent disease. Yet less than 20 percent of all Americans eat even the minimum number of fruits and vegetables suggested by nutrition experts. Hardly anybody, it seems, can work the five to seven recommended servings a day into their diet.

But juicing makes it easy. Depending upon how it's made, a single glass of juice can contain eight or more servings.

Juicing first gained fans back in the sixties as people began to realize the healthful advantages of organically grown foods. But as scientists uncovered the plethora of anticancer agents naturally found in fruits and vegetables, juicing's popularity has grown. Today, freshly squeezed juices can be found in juice bars, health clubs, and restaurants and electric juicers have become nearly as familiar a sight in home kitchens as toasters.

It isn't just freshly squeezed orange juice that people are making. Among other concoctions, they're using combinations of blueberries, ginger root, and green grapes to help battle motion sickness and a combination of parsley, spinach, grapes, and apples to stop their skin from itching. Other elixirs are used to heal urinary tract infections, ulcers, allergies, and yeast infections; reduce blood pressure; and improve skin clarity, according to many proponents.

Although both fiber and several valuable nutrients such as bioflavenoids are lost when you remove the pulp of fruits and vegetables, juicing creates an easily digestible liquid that frequently encourages people to increase their consumption of produce. While it would take some effort to eat six whole carrots and four whole stalks of celery two to three times a day, for example, the juicing process makes it as easy as sipping a glass of ice tea.

There are two ways that juice therapy is usually used: as a supplement to a full, normal diet or as part of a fast in which you eat no solid foods but consume gallons of juice and water. Keep in mind that you should always consult a physician prior to starting a juice fast—especially if you are hypoglycemic, pregnant, or diabetic, or have allergies to any foods. An unsupervised fast can be dangerous to your health and is not recommended for children under 18.

However you use juicing, you'll need to purchase a juicer, unless you're fortunate enough to live next door to a health food restaurant that is willing to custom-make your drinks.

Why can't you use canned or store-bought juices? Juicers say that the process of canning and bottling juices involves vigorous cleaning and heating that destroy many of the nutrients that make fruits and vegetables so healthful.

Fortunately, there are more and more food shops that are stocking fresh juices, and many of these juices are made from organically grown produce. But because these juices are preservative-free, they have a relatively short shelf life. So to maximize their health value, drink them as close to the purchase date as possible. You won't be alone: John Kennedy, Jr., Steven Spielberg, Alec Baldwin, Kim Basinger, Christy Brinkley, Donna Karan, and Barbra Streisand have all been known to juice.

If you decide to go on a juice fast, keep in mind four things: You must always dilute the fruit juices you make, you must drink eight or more glasses of water a day, you must limit the fast to only a few days unless under medical supervision, and you shouldn't be surprised if you don't feel well. Most people—especially those coming off a heavy diet filled with red meat and sugar—complain of headaches and sluggishness on a juice fast. Engaging in light activity may help deal with the pain of a headache. A mineral salt bath may help relax your body and mind as well. Try using a body brush to stimulate your skin prior to the bath. This may help your body to release toxins through increased surface circulation and removal of dead surface skin cells.

Remember to break all fasts with simple foods. You don't want to go from five days of juice to a steak dinner. This can catapult your digestive system into a violent turmoil that will send you hotfooting it to the nearest bathroom. Start with some broth and steamed vegetables, then gradually move back into a moderate diet over the next few days.

Fasting is an excellent way to jump-start a diet, but it's not a weight-loss regimen. After less than a week on any fast, the body starts to break down lean muscle—including the heart. So while many fasters report dropping weight fairly quickly with a juicing program, fasters are cautioned not to use juicing as a diet plan. Many fasters believe three to four short fasts a year will help keep the body healthy.

So next time you wake up with tired, gray skin and bags under your eyes, skip the hamburgers, buy yourself a book on juicing, borrow a machine, and spend a day or two juicing. It will provide the same healthful glow as expensive creams and makeup—but from the inside out.

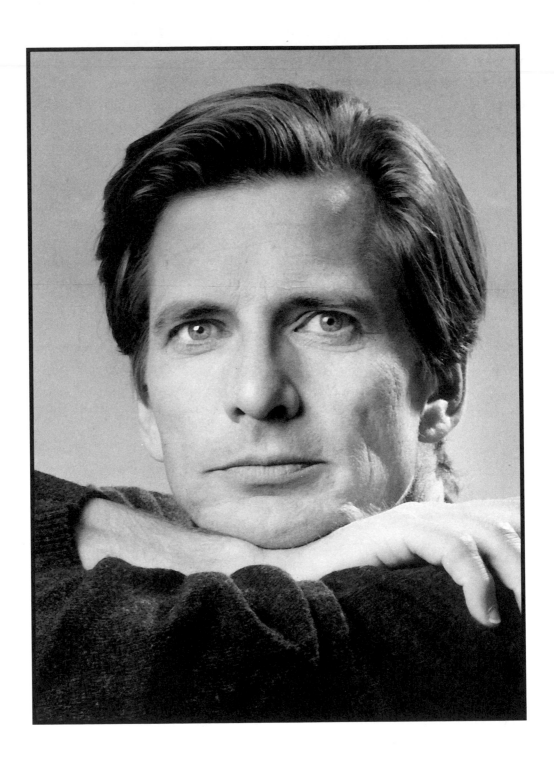

10 MACROBIOTICS

BORN
1945, White Sulfur Springs,
Montana

EDUCATION
B.A., Whitman College
(football scholarship)

CAREER HIGHLIGHTS
TELEVISION
"The A-Team"
"Battlestar Galactica"

THEATER
Butterflies Are Free (Broadway)
Abelard and Heloise (Broadway)

BOOKS
Confessions of a Kamikaze Cowboy
(an autobiography of a
journey to health)
And Then We Went Fishing

FILM
Alaska
Georgia, Georgia

"To make this work, I knew I couldn't cheat in any way. I had to change my food, my thoughts, my lifestyle, the people I associated with, the kinds of relationships I had, the way I thought about people, the kind of career I chose, and the reasons why I chose it. It was all part of the healing process."

Twenty years ago, actor Dirk Benedict stepped out of his home in Manhattan Beach, California, and wondered whether he'd be alive the following year.

"It was a very cold and gray day in April," Dirk recalls. "I walked out onto the beach with a cup of coffee in my hand, looking out at the ocean. There was hardly anyone there, and I remember thinking that my career was on a roll. I'd done a television series and a couple of movies, and I had a good social life. Basically, I had a life I didn't want to let go of."

But Dirk had just been diagnosed with prostate cancer, the third leading cause of death in men. At age thirty, not having a life to let go of was suddenly a distinct possibility.

"I was so young," says Dirk. "I felt, I suppose, what somebody feels when they're going to climb a mountain or sail across the ocean by themselves. It was a feeling of excitement and fear—and maybe a little bit of self-pity."

THE KAMIKAZE COWBOY

At first glance, Dirk is one of the last people you'd expect to be diagnosed with cancer. Raised on a ranch in Montana, he spent his early years feasting on mountain air and a steady diet of hard work, athletics, and three square meals a day.

But it was those meals high in saturated fat, cholesterol, refined sugar, and carbohydrates that Dirk believes set the stage for the drama of his cancer. "Breakfast was steak and eggs, ham and eggs, hash browns, pancakes, and hot cereal—usually all at the same time. I ate meat at every meal—mostly wild meat like deer, elk, pheasant, and some trout," says the actor. What did he wash it down with? "Beer, and lots of it," he replies.

These eating and drinking habits continued into college. "In my college fraternity I held the record for eating sloppy joes—twenty-four," says Dirk with a mischievous grin.

By the time Dirk's cancer test came back positive, he already knew there was a problem with his prostate. "I had been having prostate problems on and off since I was sixteen or seventeen," he explains. "Somewhere around a year prior to my official diagnosis, my prostate became enlarged, and I had been having varying degrees of pain while urinating.

"It made me apprehensive approaching a bathroom," he adds. "I never knew exactly what would happen. There would be a burning sensation when I urinated that made me grab on to whatever was closest for support. Then came the day when I found blood in my urine."

To his doctor, Dirk's next step was obvious—check into the nearest hospital immediately for surgery. But Dirk wasn't so sure. He thanked the doctor for his opinion, then went back home to walk on the beach.

The problem was that no one knew what had caused the cancer. Nor did anyone have a treatment that was guaranteed. Because although surgery today has a 93 percent success rate when prostate cancer is detected early and before the onset of any symptoms of the disease, many of the tests, surgical techniques, and follow-up therapies that contribute to that rate were not developed until a decade or more after Dirk had been diagnosed, unfortunately.

Faced with a scientific community that couldn't guarantee success and warned of some substantial side effects—impotence or castration were two potential risks—Dirk turned his back on conventional medicine. Instead of surgery, he opted to make a total, wholehearted commitment to a macrobiotic lifestyle—an Oriental way of living based on the philosophy that health and happiness are achieved when we live in harmony with the natural laws of the universe. All he had read about macrobiotics as a way to combat cancer made total sense and held more hope for him than the odds of going through the conventional treatments.

NATURAL EATING

Nowhere else is the macrobiotic approach more evident in the lives of its adherents than in diet. Fifty percent of the macrobiotic diet is whole grains like brown rice, wheat noodles, barley, oats, or buckwheat; 30 percent is cooked vegetables; 15 percent is cooked beans; and 5 percent is miso soup. It sounds fairly simple. But within each of these food groups, individual foods are assigned specific values that must be carefully balanced. Complicating that task is the necessity for the individual to evaluate each food in terms of whether eating it will promote harmony.

"I had been studying macrobiotic philosophy for three years," says Dirk. "I had quit eating sugar, and I was avoiding chemicals. But the body does not regenerate or rejuvenate overnight, and my prostate problems had already been there for a long time. So I figured the journey back would take nearly as long—six to eight years—for the prostate to go back to normal."

Dirk had first been introduced to macrobiotics when he starred on Broadway with screen idol Gloria Swanson in the play *Butterflies Are Free*.

"One night Gloria invited me to her home for dinner and stepped out of her movie-star role and into an apron," Dirk recalls. She rustled up a genuine macrobiotic meal for Dirk and her husband, William Duffy, that included corn chowder, rice cakes with tahini, and bancha tea.

Dirk was intrigued. Since he left Montana, he had already given up refined sugar, white bread, soda pop, and meat. But the macrobiotic approach piqued his curiosity, and he began to integrate some of its principles into his diet. As his eating changed, so did his body. For instance, he lost the arthritic pain in his knees that had been with him since his late teens.

Dirk established a daily routine that enabled him to begin a macrobiotic lifestyle. He rose early before filming each day to fix a breakfast of miso soup and oatmeal, and a lunch of brown rice and vegetables to take along with him to the set.

"But I wasn't yet totally macrobiotic," says Dirk. "I had quit eating animal protein. And I didn't eat eggs, meat, or chicken. But I still ate fish, I still drank coffee, I put milk in it, and if I was in a vegetarian restaurant and cheese was put on my food, I ate it."

But the cancer diagnosis changed Dirk's diet forever. "I knew that, let's say, putting one pat of butter on a bagel once every four months could be the difference between surviving and not surviving," says Dirk. "So to make this work, I knew I couldn't cheat in any way. I had to change my food, my thoughts, my lifestyle, the people I associated with, the kinds of relationships I had, the way I thought about people, the kind of career I chose, and the reasons why I chose it. It was all part of the healing process.

"But once I decided to go that route, I never once went back on my decision," Dirk adds. "I knew the statistics with regard to prostate cancer, and I didn't want to risk it. It was just a question of whether I had the spiritual fortitude to stick with it—that I wasn't so sure about."

Dirk spoke with Michio Kushi, a master teacher of macrobiotics, who confirmed what Dirk had come to know—that even cancer could be a friend if it led to enlightenment. Kushi then loaned Dirk the use of his mountain cabin in New Hampshire to help him find it.

THE GREAT ESCAPE

Kushi's cabin represented much more than a place to stay. For Dirk it would be the hideaway he needed to reorder his life and begin his recovery. Taking little more than macrobiotic groceries and a toothbrush, Dirk fled to the mountains.

"It was a deserted community with just a couple of cabins," recalls Dirk. "But to me it was like the Garden of Eden."

Left alone without books or television or even a picture on the wall to distract him, Dirk prayed, meditated, and concentrated on getting better. It was his transformation in this cabin that Dirk would soon be writing about in his autobiography, *Confessions of a Kamikaze Cowboy*, the chronicle of his journey from cancer victim to survivor.

"I took walks through the forest and thought about all my relationships and my childhood," says the actor. "I would talk to the animals and the trees and the birds. All the while, I was going through these experiences where my body would be physically discharging stuff that had been stored away for years. Sometimes, it was very painful."

During his time in the mountains, Dirk ate a macrobiotic diet of 80 percent whole grains and 20 percent vegetables. He drank only water or non-stimulating teas. Everything he ate was cooked—nothing was raw, not even the vegetables. It was all either steamed, boiled, or pressure-cooked.

"I also paid attention to how I ate—never overeating and making sure to chew each bite at least 150 times," adds Dirk.

Six weeks later, Dirk emerged from the cabin, a changed man—and thirty pounds lighter.

LIGHTS, CAMERA, ACTION

Dirk traveled and allowed his body to continue healing. At one point, "I went to see my sister—who didn't know I had cancer—and she didn't recognize me," recounts Dirk. "I said, 'Ramona,' and she turned, screamed, and started sobbing. I looked like somebody who was in the final stages of cancer, except I had this buoyant spirit."

That spirit kept him going even through the inevitable feelings of is-this-really-working, until Hollywood distracted him with the deal he couldn't refuse: a starring role in the new TV series "Battlestar Galactica."

But first, there was the studio physical. When the doctor queried Dirk about any preexisting physical problems, Dirk lied, believing they would never understand how he had been curing himself of cancer. And he passed the physical with flying colors.

"Battlestar Galactica" became a big hit, which led to his next project two seasons later, the mega-hot TV series "The A-Team," in which Dirk was cast—along with Mr. T—as the beautiful face on the show. But this time the physical didn't go exactly as Dirk had planned. Although he easily passed an exam that decreed him healthy and insurable, someone had tipped off the insurance company that Dirk had been battling cancer, and the doctor wanted to talk about it. Fortunately, Dirk had passed a test for prostate cancer several months before and could assure the doctor that cancer was in his past—not his future.

Today Dirk is both an attentive father and a busy actor preparing for his next film, a starring role that will take him on location to Alaska. And even though this hunky actor has just turned fifty, he will be playing the role of a man ten years his junior—one of the advantages of embracing a diet that keeps you young. Although, as Dirk is always careful to remind friends, "for me, macrobiotics is a way of life—not just a diet."

SPOTLIGHT ON MACROBIOTICS

If you believe life is frozen food cooked for three minutes in a microwave and wolfed down in front of the TV set, a macrobiotic lifestyle may be hard for you to swallow. But if you're ready to marvel at nature and appreciate every bite of the food you're eating, you may be a prime candidate for this ancient discipline.

To those who place a high priority on the ease and convenience of fast food like a pizza from the local trattoria, becoming a "brown rice junkie" who eats organically grown unprocessed foods may appear to be just too much trouble. But to the millions worldwide who wouldn't think of living any other way, this way of eating and being has come to represent the means to a happier, healthier, and more productive life.

Macrobiotics, which literally translates to "larger life," is based on the idea that health and happiness are the product of living in harmony with the natural laws of the universe. These laws, according to macrobiotic teaching, are governed by the following seven principles:

Everything is a difference of one infinity—we come from one source.

Everything changes.

All antagonisms are complementary.

There is nothing identical.

What has a front has a back.

The bigger the front, the bigger the back.

What has a beginning has an end.

While reading this list won't instantly grant you a balanced life, adherents to macrobiotics believe that by exploring these principles through contemplation and action, they can begin to understand how these principles exist within all things, from the thoughts they think to the food they consume. They also believe that when consciously applied to their lives—through diet, prayer, and meditation, for example—these principles will allow them to create a life free from illness and full of health.

The key to applying these principles is to live a life that balances "yin" and "yang," two forces that represent polar opposites in Eastern thought. In diet, for example, foods that are considered "too yin" or "too yang" can cause illness. Foods that are balanced between the two extremes can cure illness.

Highly yin foods such as sugar, most fruit, dairy products, oil, alcohol, coffee, sweets, potatoes, tomatoes, and spices are totally eliminated from a macrobiotic diet, as are foods that are overly yang—meat, eggs, cheese, and poultry. One exception is fish consumed on an infrequent basis.

Does it all seem a bit "out there"? Although there is no scientific basis for the notion that a macrobiotic diet can heal, there is scientific basis for the concepts of yin and yang. These two polarities correlate to the acid-base measurement of food, which is why food normally found to be high in either of these two substances is not allowed in a macrobiotic diet. Just as the pH-balanced shampoo you may be using claims to create healthier hair, macrobiotics claims that eating pH-balanced food will translate into greater overall health.

The pH scale runs from 0 to 14, with 1 being the most yang, 14 the most yin, and 7 neutral or "balanced." Brown rice, a staple in all macrobiotic diets, is a 7. Food between 0 and 7 is considered highly acidic or yang. Food between 7 and 14 is highly alkaline and yin.

A balanced diet in macrobiotic terms is composed of 50 percent or more whole cereal grains like brown rice, whole wheat, wheat noodles, barley, oats, oatmeal, corn, and buckwheat; 30 percent cooked vegetables; 15 percent cooked beans such as adzuki beans, chickpeas, lentils, or black beans; and the remaining 5 percent miso soup.

Although there is a basic macrobiotic diet, many other factors—including time of year, where you live, and your lifestyle—are taken into consideration when determining the exact diet for you. Much of this can be learned on your own by reading books on the subject. But as you begin to think in terms of yin and yang, you will see that many of your natural instincts are encouraging you to balance yin and yang.

Have you ever noticed how you feel the need to follow your salty hamburger with a sweet soda? That's your natural way of trying to balance the yin and yang qualities of food. People who embrace macrobiotics follow this line of reasoning through even to whom they choose to be with in a relationship. A strongly yin person will look for someone with dominant yang qualities to provide a balanced relationship.

And you thought macrobiotics was about nothing but a bowl of brown rice?

Macrobiotics was practiced only in Japan by a small group of people until George Ohsawa brought it to the United States in the 1950s. Ohsawa, who blamed chronic illness during his young adulthood on the Western diet adopted by his parents, had essentially developed the concept as an amalgam of Oriental medicine and its associated cosmology. It had healed him, and he believed it could heal the world. After Ohsawa's death in 1966, his student Michio Kushi set up centers dedicated to teaching the underlying principles of macrobiotics. Schools, restaurants, and even supermarkets dedicated to a macrobiotic way of living began to pop up throughout the United States.

Common sense dictates that you should check with your physician before going on any radical diet such as macrobiotics, especially when considering a macrobiotic diet for children in their developmental years. But for the thousands of people who have embraced a macrobiotic way of life to create harmony and health among body, mind, and spirit, it works.

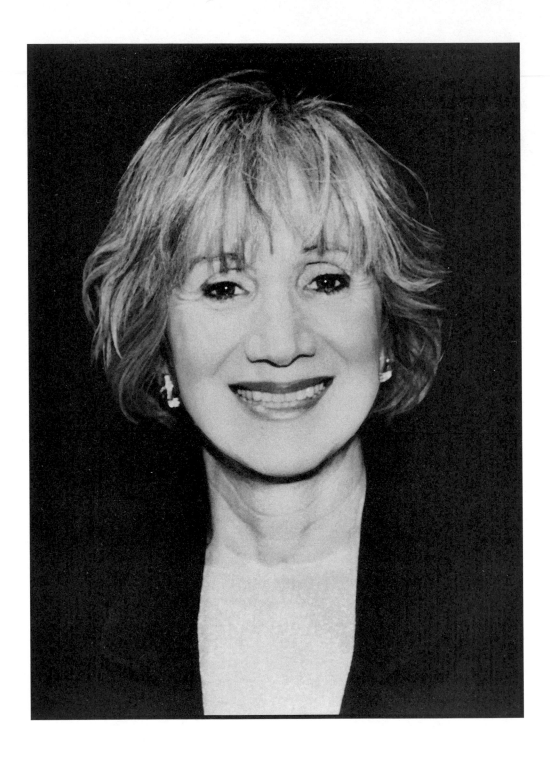

11 MASSAGE THERAPY

BORN
Lowell, Massachusetts

PROFESSIONAL AWARDS
Academy Award,
Best Supporting Actress:
Moonstruck
New York Film Critics Award:
Moonstruck
Los Angeles Film Critics Award:
Moonstruck
Golden Globe Award: *Moonstruck*
ACE Award: *The Last Act Is A Solo*
Obie Awards: *A Man's A Man* and
The Marriage of Bette and Boo

CAREER HIGHLIGHTS
THEATER
Social Security
The Curse of the Starving Class

FILM
Mr. Holland's Opus
The Cemetery Club
Steel Magnolias
Look Who's Talking

TELEVISION
"Tales of the City"
"Young at Heart"
"A Century of Women"

"Anytime you're able to experience something cathartic in which you're able to reclaim yourself, you're creating an environment for health."

Whether you see her accepting a rose from Frank Sinatra in a made-for-TV movie, stealing scenes from Shirley MacLaine on the big screen, or having the time of her life whirling across a stage, audiences have come to expect a lot from Academy Award–winning actress Olympia Dukakis.

And they should. At sixty-something, Olympia has more than proven her talent and professional expertise as an actress, producer, director, teacher, even political campaigner. Who can forget her impassioned speeches on behalf of her cousin Michael's bid for the presidency?

Even though Olympia appears completely secure with whatever role she plays, there's another side to this magnificent woman that is less assured. In fact, underneath the professional polish, Olympia deals with issues often associated with self-worth.

"I had a lot of low self-esteem from the start," Olympia candidly admits. "Part of it came from being Greek. I think that there are minorities all over who have it. Jewish women, black women—we all have it. The world is busy telling us that we're less than who we really are and we don't quite understand why.

"Like most women, I got hit with it during my teenage years," adds Olympia. "And that takes many years to shovel yourself out of."

The going was tough, but Olympia was not only tough, she was smart. "When I realized that I was going to be hamstrung for my ethnicity, I decided to start a theater," she explains. Thumbing her nose at traditional outlets for her talent, she made her own opportunities. In fact, by using her own theater as a learning lab, she developed her skills not only as an actress but as a producer and director as well, and then went on to share them as a graduate school instructor at New York University.

Then she got that "lucky break."

"I did a play called *Social Security* at the same time that director Norman Jewison was trying to cast the movie *Moonstruck*," Olympia says. Jewison saw Olympia's potential and cast her in a major role. Before long, Olympia was picking up an Oscar for Best Supporting Actress.

You might have thought this would have wiped away any of Olympia's self-doubt, but it didn't. "I'm a human being and we all have these feelings," says the actress with a laugh. "I'm not surprised that at times I feel helpless, hopeless, and fragile. These feelings don't just go away because you've succeeded in something."

On the other hand, she adds, "that doesn't mean they have to control your life."

OLYMPIA'S ADVENTURE

Olympia realized from the start of her acting career that the way to keep any feelings of helplessness or fragility under control was to give them the attention they deserved. She found several ways to do this, but in true Olympia style, she found one that was truly unique: massage.

Massage is a form of bodywork generally reserved for those who want to relieve muscle aches and pains or increase circulation. But Olympia saw it as an opportunity to work with her feelings and pamper herself in the process. An "I am worth this time and money" session on a massage table is guaranteed to send healing messages to even the most wounded psyche. "The last person most of us think about is ourselves," says Olympia. "But sometime, someplace, you have to stop and say you're worthwhile."

How did Olympia find a massage therapist? "I was conducting a workshop at a retreat center in Upstate New York," recalls Olympia. "While I was there, I met a woman who was leading a workshop on bodywork. Every once in a while she would come up to me and put her hand on my back, and I would feel something happening. She didn't talk or say anything, but I was aware that her hand was not like the hand of an ordinary person. I thought, 'This is an extraordinary woman, and I want to know her.'"

The woman was Ilana Rubenfeld, the creator of Rubenfeld Synergy, a combination of several forms of massage with an active listening technique that its developer feels helps integrate mind and body.

Meeting Ilana was enough for Olympia to know that she wanted to experience Ilana's special form of bodywork, which practitioners say is helpful in identifying, expressing, and working through deep feelings and memories that may be locked away in the body.

The opportunity came a few weeks later at Ilana's massage school in Greenwich Village, New York, a stone's throw from Olympia's New Jersey home. "I wasn't in pain or in need," Olympia says, "but I wanted to use the work as a wonderful kind of adventure to find out more about what the hell is inside of me."

Ilana led Olympia into a treatment room on the second floor of her six-story brownstone. She dimmed the lights, put on soft music, and set up a massage table. Olympia prepared herself by removing her shoes, jewelry, belt, and bra, opting for a minimum amount of loose-fitting clothing. She got up on the table and Ilana began her work.

Although treatments differ according to the needs of the client, the synergist—the name given to a bodyworker who performs the Rubenfeld technique—usually begins by touching the head very gently to first establish contact to let the client know that the session has begun and the synergist is listening. During these initial movements, a bond of trust begins to grow between the two.

The synergist then moves on to lightly palpate the muscles. This is a technique that allows bodyworkers to "listen" through their hands for any traumas the body might be holding on to, as indicated by tenseness in the muscles. When a tense area is found, the synergist will massage the area, but may also verbally point it out so that the client can begin to recognize what tension feels like within the body and then take part in its release.

Olympia and Ilana exchanged few words. Instead Ilana did most of her communication through her hands, occasionally asking Olympia about areas where her muscles seemed especially tense.

Slowly Olympia began to identify the origins of some of the tenseness Ilana found and, by acknowledging it, began to let it go. "I found myself getting in touch with all those things that I had bottled up or denied," says the actress. "I ended up laughing and crying and even getting scared."

Scared? Olympia Dukakis?

"You get scared because the work becomes very in-depth," explains Olympia. "All of the things we have experienced in our lives are in our bodies. We think they are only on tape in our heads because we like to think of ourselves as rational human beings. But the entire body is really a tape. The knee has experienced what the knee was involved with, for example, so if you can really get into the knee and work with the knee, things are going to be released."

How do these experiences get released?

Mostly through talking, says Olympia. "I found myself talking when Ilana asked me something or I felt like it. Sometimes she would touch a specific part of my body, like a shoulder, and ask what was going on there." Using gestalt therapy, a psychological process where the client is asked to talk to parts of their body as if these parts could respond to them, the client may be asked to address the wrist, or hip, or spine to find out more about what is going on inside. The synergist gently guides the client into this by asking open-ended questions. As the synergists touch and massage, they question—

either verbally or through their hands—tell me what is happening right here in your body?

"What I did was tell her what my body was feeling both emotionally and physically," says Olympia. "I told her, 'I feel uncomfortable, I feel frightened.' But it was clear that she knew, that what I was describing from a physical standpoint was another language that has to do with who you are and the impact of experiences that you've had in your life—the fears, the hopes, and the dreams that you carry around with you in the present. You don't get scared because they touch you. You get scared because their work becomes very in-depth and things are going to get released."

Olympia wasn't sure if there was an exact incident that was triggering her feelings, "but that's not what's really important," she says. "What's important is to claim the feelings that came up as part of you. With this work I was able to claim what was there—my rage, my childishness, my maturity, my romanticism, my realism—all my humanity. It's all about claiming who you are, and being more who you are makes your life more vibrant.

"By the time I got up off the table," adds Olympia, "I felt less defensive. My heart was right out there, and I knew I was more available to people. I felt like I could look at people, and talk with them without feeling any distance." As a wife and mother, Olympia finds this especially rewarding.

"When we do these things, we acknowledge all parts of ourselves, even the part that feels defeated at times," adds Olympia. "We, especially women, live in a lot of silence—feeling [that] our voice isn't worth anything, or that our bodies are truly valuable only in a physical sense."

"As a result, I am more open and vulnerable. I don't feel as if I need or want anything. I become more real and more honest. It brings better relationships," says Olympia.

As an actress, Olympia finds this invaluable. "I want my plateful of whatever life is. As this translates into my work, I permit more to happen and I'm less on guard," she says. "And anytime [you're] able to experience something cathartic in which you're able to reclaim yourself, you're then creating an environment for health."

Ultimately, that's why massage can be so therapeutic. "I think it goes beyond medical; it goes to the spirit. It permits a deeper integration between my thoughts, my feelings and my body," says Olympia. "And that brings clarity and healing."

SPOTLIGHT ON MASSAGE

If your image of massage is husky Joe from the local gym throwing you down on a hard table to pound away at sore and aching muscles—it's time to rethink this therapy. Ditto for the celluloid fable of massage being solely for the rich and bored. Because today, bodywork—the name given to everything from movement awareness to Swedish massage—has graduated to a therapeutic art form that has millions diving for the nearest massage table as they gently give over to its healing virtues.

The real story on bodywork began in ancient Greece, where soldiers returning from the battlefield were met with a hearty meal and a massage. About the same time these guys were laying their bodies down for a postwar pick-me-up, their neighbors in the Orient were busy developing their own method of massage called Shiatsu. Soon Oriental therapists were running their fingers along energy pathways that travel throughout the body in an effort to locate and release any tension.

Today, bodywork is an evolving field that has come to encompass a host of new practices, all of which work to relieve tension and stress, relax the body, and open the paths for the body's own healing energies to flow through.

In *Swedish Massage*, the masseuse uses long, gliding strokes to enhance circulation, the kneading of individual muscles to enhance relaxation, and a tapping movement to energize nerves.

In the *Trager Method*, the practitioner cradles and moves the various limbs by rocking and shaking the joints, all in an effort to stimulate the production of joint fluid, a substance that Trager practitioners believe helps diseases pass through the body.

In the *Alexander Technique*, practitioners use a light, buoyant touch to guide the client, actually thought of as a student, into more efficient directions of movement. The technique was developed by an actor, F. Matthias Alexander, who used it to eliminate vocal problems he was having. He felt that the way gravity affects people—making the head slump forward—puts a strain on their bodies. His solution was to retrain the body to be lighter, mostly by becoming aware of habitual patterns like slumping.

In *Rubenfeld Synergy*, the synergist uses both constant touch and an active listening technique to elicit memories and encourage integration and healing of both body and mind.

Whichever form of massage you choose, you'll be hard-pressed to find a more soothing and nurturing way to spend an hour or two of your time. A good way to begin is with a simple massage in which the muscles and soft tissues are gently kneaded and manipulated in an effort to reduce pain, alleviate stress, and improve overall health.

Once thought of as an outrageous luxury saved for James Bond and the royal family, a massage has become as common as a haircut. Most sessions range anywhere from $30 to $200, depending on the type of work you choose, length of the session, and any special extras, such as two practitioners synchronistically working your body, or scented oils imported from India or the Orient with which to anoint your body.

Many forms of bodywork require rigorous training and certification. But keep in mind that because not all states have licensing requirements—no licensing is required in over two-thirds of the country—almost anybody with a minimum of experience can hang out a shingle.

So before booking an appointment, consider getting a recommendation from someone you know and trust. Given the intimate nature of this therapy, you'll want to know in whose hands you've placed your body. Reputable massage therapists have a strict code of ethics that stresses modesty; neither genitalia nor female breasts are exposed.

After the massage begins, don't be afraid to tell the bodyworker how gently or firmly you want them to work. And, of course, tell them of any preexisting medical conditions, especially recent surgery, skin disorders, diabetes, high blood pressure, cardiovascular disease, or allergies.

Don't limit your massage to times of tension and stress. Many office workers report a ten-minute massage break during lunch has them returning to their desk physically invigorated and mentally alert and ready to tackle the rest of the day.

But to turn your simple massage into a mini vacation, get the massage as late in the day as possible. Many practitioners work at night and weekends so that you have time to relax and luxuriate in the afterglow of a good massage. Choose your favorite music to play in the background, lower the lights, and consider taking a warm bath to prepare your body to really absorb the experience.

While Swedish massage leaves you pleasantly sleepy, many report that Shiatsu gets you up and ready for a vigorous day of activity, while Trager and Rubenfeld leave you in an open and vulnerable place with a pleasantly spacey feeling. Keep all this in consideration when booking an appointment.

The fastest and most cost-effective way to start is by picking up a bottle of massage oil on your way home from the office tonight and treating your partner to a head-to-foot once-over. Or if that sounds too intimidating, try a simple (but just as rewarding) hand or foot massage. Don't worry about technique—there's enough medical research to suggest that the loving touch of a significant other is enough to spark our internal healing energies.

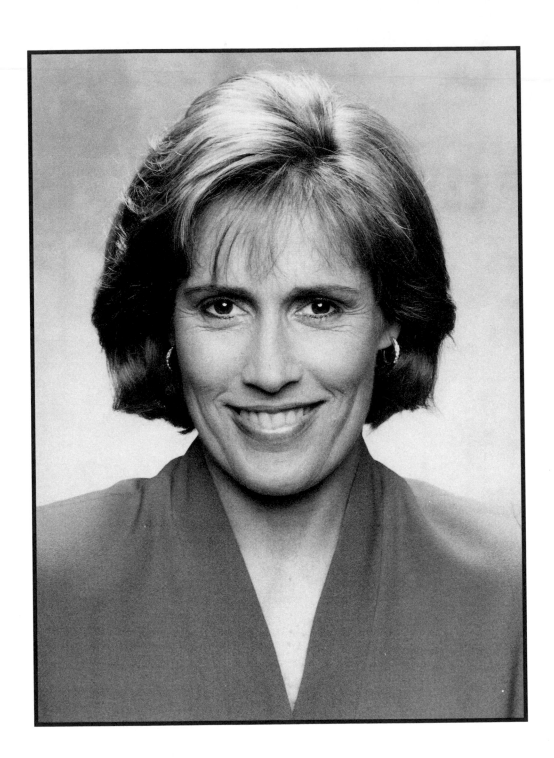

12 MIND/BODY MEDICINE

BORN
August 22, 1950,
Southern California

EDUCATION
Lake Forest College,
Phi Betta Kappa

CAREER HIGHLIGHTS
World record for the longest
swim by man or woman
(from Bahamas to Florida),
102.5 miles, set in 1979

TV correspondent and segment
producer, "The Crusaders"

Host, "America's Vital Signs,"
a health show on CNBC

"One on One with Diana Nyad,"
a TV interview series

Announcer, "ABC's Wide World
of Sports"

Entertainment reporter, CBS
News—San Francisco

Radio commentator, National
Public Radio's "Morning Edition"

BOOKS
*The Philosophy of Extremism, Basic
Training and Other Shores*

*"It's not that you make this mind/body connection
and all your health problems go away. But, as I
learn to slow down, listen to my body, and breathe
deeply, I find this approach really is working for
me."*

In 1978, a disheartened Diana Nyad emerged
from the water. An attempt at a record-breaking
swim from Cuba to Florida had failed. With her
nearly unstoppable will still urging her on, Diana
was forced onto dry land by impossible weather
conditions and innumerable jellyfish stings.

There wasn't a newspaper in the Western
world that didn't feature Diana's swollen and
exhausted body as front-page news, speculating
that the swimmer, who left the water some
twenty-nine pounds thinner, would soon be
retiring.

"I was pretty beaten up," recalls Diana. "I'd
had enough of this sport; it's a tough grind, and
I was whipped. I had just spent a year training for
that swim. I thought to myself, 'I have other tal-
ents and it's time for me to move on.'"

But like a prizefighter knocked out for the
count, only to return to the ring weeks later, ego

and drive intact, Diana began to imagine what it would be like to give it one last try, even as she recuperated.

"After a couple of days on IVs in the hospital, I started to feel a little better and realized that it was more the fault of the weather than me or my crew that had gotten in the way of my reaching shore. I started dreaming of once again making the swim. Slowly, I started to get it together."

Within weeks Diana was ready to start training again. But this time, the stakes would be even higher. "I decided I wasn't going to quit this sport until I had the big one, the unprecedented, unbeatable, ego trip, long-distance swim."

In August 1978, almost one year later, a twenty-nine-year-old Diana entered the waters of the Bahamas, heading for Florida in an attempt to make the longest swim ever, 102 miles. A thirty-year-old Diana emerged two days later with the world's record for the longest swim in history—for either man or woman—a title she still holds.

True to her word, Diana left swimming and transferred her passion to a new career, broadcasting. She attacked this with the same fervor, and it's safe to say that for years nothing could slow Diana Nyad to a crawl; at least, nothing could until a bout with allergies nearly shut off her breathing and got in the way of her lucrative broadcasting career.

It happened when Diane was on vacation in Mexico. Her throat began to swell so frighteningly that she was raced to a hospital just over the border in San Diego. There doctors found that polyps they believed were caused by the allergies had swollen until they were obstructing her airway. The doctors reduced the swelling so she could breathe, then discharged her from the hospital with the recommendation that she see a specialist at Cedars–Sinai Medical Center in Los Angeles who could remove the polyps.

Diana did, and the specialist recommended immediate surgery.

But Diana was unimpressed by the doctor's urgency. "I was working as a local anchor in San Francisco," explains Diana. "I told the doctor at Cedars–Sinai that I'd get the operation sometime soon, but that I had to get back to work.

"He said, 'You're crazy. If this happens again, and you can't get to a hospital fast enough, your throat will swell to the point where you won't be able to breathe.'"

Diana finally agreed, and polyps were removed from her throat, vocal cords, sinuses, and nasal passages.

The surgery gave Diana room to breathe, literally and figuratively, and she used the time recuperating to think about how she had developed the allergies, what aggravated them, and how, once and for all, they might be either eliminated or at least brought under control. Otherwise, she realized, more polyps might grow and she'd be right back in the same hospital bed in the not-too-distant future.

"My allergies began in Italy in 1975. The day before, I had had a race from the Isle of Capri to Naples. I had won it many times. Besides swimming in warm water, which is great, Italians are so passionate that I loved that race. But the morning after the race, I woke up with a heavy cold, which isn't unusual for a swimmer, given the number of hours you spend in the water and how it affects you. You become a little peaked, lose weight, and experience a bit of an immune system depression."

But the "cold" never left. "Over the years I used many things to cure this 'cold,' which was really allergies. I saw immunologists who want you there every day of the week for treatment. I had all the immunization shots, which if you are lucky, cure 20 percent of the problem. But given how many allergies I have, it's crazy to take all those shots. At that time, I was also traveling a lot, so for two years I actually gave myself those shots. They never really helped."

As a swimmer, "I needed to be able to breathe freely, so I was also taking injections of a steroid used to shrink back tissue," says Diana. "I would get all the oxygen I needed, but I knew continued use of steroids is very dangerous. You can start to swell up, have liver problems or even heart problems. I was scared to death about taking them."

While swimming, Diana was reluctant to try an alternative method, preferring to stick with a technique she knew. But, stuck in the hospital and recovering from surgery, Diana began to look for other ways to deal with the allergies and the polyps that could someday grow back. What she eventually discovered was mind/body medicine.

THE HEALER WITHIN

Those who practice mind/body medicine believe that the body has the innate capacity to heal itself. The individual's object is to discover what stresses, both physical and emotional, are contributing to the illness, and to use therapies such as biofeedback, hypnotherapy, meditation, relaxation, deep breathing, massage, and yoga to counteract those stresses and help the body heal itself.

Her first step was to identify any stresses that were contributing to her allergies. There were two, Diana acknowledges. The first was her tendency always to be in a hurry. "My philosophy had always been, 'How much can I accomplish, given how little time I have?' " says Diana. "I remember at ten being asked what I wanted to be when I grew up. All I could think about was that my grandmother had died at eighty-two and, whatever I chose, I only had seventy-two years to do it in!" What's more, Diana's last thought before going to sleep as a child, was how much time she would be forced to sleep before she could get up.

This sense of urgency was a driving stressor in her life. But as fast as her sense of urgency drove her forward, another stressor was holding her back: sexual abuse.

It's not something she likes to dwell on, but Diana tells the story candidly: By the time her eighteenth birthday rolled around, she was ready for the 1968 Olympic tryouts. But as hard as Diana tried, she failed to make the team. "Two things happened that year at the trials," explains the athlete. "I had passed my speed peak. And, after years of being sexually abused by my swimming coach, I had lost my confidence. By the time I got to the trials, I was feeling terribly alone and confused, and abuse was part of it.

"I believe this is why I chose marathon swimming and stayed with it for ten years," she adds. "In the ocean, I could totally escape. I was immersed for eight to ten hours at a time and nobody could get to me. They couldn't even talk to me."

Now, years later, lying alone in her hospital bed, recovering from polyp surgery, Diana got in touch with how her past was affecting her health.

"I realized that I had to go beyond the symptoms of my allergies, and beyond what was left over from my years of sexual abuse," says the athlete.

Conversations with doctors and reading helped Diana learn just how important the mind/body connection could be in restoring health.

"I started reading books like *Siddhartha* that introduced me to a whole new way of looking at life," she says. "Sometimes I found that just talking about pressures I was feeling helped me to breathe better. I was beginning to see that I could be happy and calm, rather than always racing."

Diana decided to use two of mind/body medicine's most potent techniques, relaxation and deep breathing, to activate her body's innate healing system. She hoped these techniques would alleviate her allergies by removing both the sense of urgency and the leftover angst that had caused such stress in her life.

"I think my Achilles' heel is in my breathing apparatus," says Diana. "But I found that taking the time to breathe in and out, and even following my breath, brought me greater calm. It allowed me to be present in the moment, and in a state of greater peace."

The breathing that Diana refers to is not just your everyday huffing and puffing. It is a technique in which an individual sits with eyes closed, feet flat on the floor, and takes a slow, deep breath, then slowly exhales with equal deliberation. The individual concentrates only on the sound and feeling of the breath entering and leaving the body.

As John Doulliard, a Colorado-based chiropractor and author of *Mind, Body, and Sport*, says, "Breath connects the mind and the body. If someone is in the fight-or-flight response"—which is how the body reacts to stress—"the tendency is for that person to stop breathing fully. This response can be brought on by stress; illness; physical, sexual, or emotional abuse; or even by an athletic quest."

"You can often identify people—especially athletes—who are experiencing this by the way they breathe through their mouths," he adds. "Breathing through the nose, which is what babies naturally do, is a basic skill talked about in many health disciplines. Taking the time to relax and breathe is a key component to anyone's health."

As Diana has come to understand this, she's learned to make herself literally stop and smell the roses.

"There's a rosebush right outside my front door," says the athlete. "Now when I see that bush, I make myself slow down. I take a deep knee bend and really put my nose in the rose and smell it. I don't think about what my life is, or what I want my life to be, or any of the do-or-die issues I tend to get caught up in. For a few seconds, I just breathe."

It's not easy for an achiever like Diana to stop her race toward the future for even a few moments. But "a few years back, I went to Thailand for the first time and read a lot about using your breath to get your mind out of the way," she says. "I'm not talking about the type of relaxation that's like falling asleep, but the kind in which I direct my thoughts to a calm place."

The reading helped, admits Diana. And today, "I know how much better I feel when I take the time to get into my backyard Jacuzzi, lie back, and look at the stars.

"As I become a more peaceful person and work on my soul part, I start to breathe and feel better. It's not that you make this mind/body connection and all your health problems go away. But, as I learn to slow down, listen to my body, and breathe deeply, I find this approach really is working for me."

SPOTLIGHT ON MIND/BODY MEDICINE

Can a cynical outlook on life really make you more susceptible to a virus? Can hating your job create more colds? How about the effects of being in a life-threatening situation—is it enough to enable a petite, 100-pound woman to leap over a ten-foot fence or lift a 500-pound boulder that happens to be in her way? Does your doctor's beliefs about your illness have an effect on your health and your body's ability to heal?

The idea that the mind affects our bodies through what we believe, our emotions, and our moods is the basis of mind/body medicine.

It's a concept that is being explored in both the traditional and alternative medical communities. Since the 1970s, medical research has begun to confirm what Eastern systems of medicine have believed for centuries—that when it comes to our body's health and illness, the mind plays a powerful role. Laboratory research has revealed that the body has naturally occurring chemicals called neuropeptides that transmit messages between the brain and cells in the nervous, endocrine, and immune systems. These messengers translate the feelings of mood, pain, pleasure, and stress into chemicals that trigger specific physical responses within the body. While a particular emotion will not in and of itself actually create illness, it can sabotage the immune system by releasing naturally occurring chemicals that will suppress the body's normal immune response—thus laying the groundwork for infectious diseases.

But there are also indications in the research that positive thoughts and emotions can also have good effects on the immune system—giving it at least a transient boost that might help fight infection.

Since the results of this groundbreaking research were made public, a running debate has taken place between scientists as to how much the mind can do. One of the landmark studies in this area was done by a physician whom many people consider the pioneer of psychoneuroimmunology, Robert Adler, M.D. He conditioned the immune systems of rats by giving them a diet of saccharin and a drug that suppressed the immune system, then took away the suppressants but continued the saccharin. The result? The rats' immune systems continued to be suppressed even though they were no longer being the fed the drug. The saccharin was enough to trigger a response. To some scientists, the inescapable conclusion was that the mind has a very specific effect upon the body's health. Dr. Adler's experiments opened up a Pandora's box of questions that have yet to be answered—including exactly how memories, thoughts, and responses to smells, tastes, touch, and myriad other stimuli could create a physical response within the body.

While many of these questions remain unanswered by medical science, clinicians are beginning to use relaxation techniques like deep breathing, biofeedback, hypnosis, meditation, and visualization in an attempt to encourage the body to boost production of the naturally occurring chemicals that might increase the number of immune system cells in the body. Radiologist O. Carl Simonton, M.D., for example, taught cancer patients how to make their bodies more receptive to radiation treatments by visualizing their cancer cells disappearing.

Perhaps the most widely accepted mind/body work is that of Dean Ornish, M.D., whose groundbreaking work in reversing heart disease through a program of diet, exercise, and meditation (a form of mind/body work used for relaxation) has been so widely accepted that some health insurance companies will even cover the costs of his program.

Generally, mind/body medicine is most effective when used together with the weapons of conventional medicine to forge an all-out offensive on a particular health problem. Most doctors who use mind/body medicine emphasize that it is an adjunct treatment. Take high blood pressure, for example. When used in conjunction with traditional blood pressure medications, deep breathing has been able to help reduce blood pressure enough in some people that the amount of medication—and its side effects—can be significantly reduced.

Tomorrow morning when you reach for your cereal, try a little mind/body technique by thinking about just how wonderful your life really is. Imagine all the terrific things in store for you and skip the worrying.

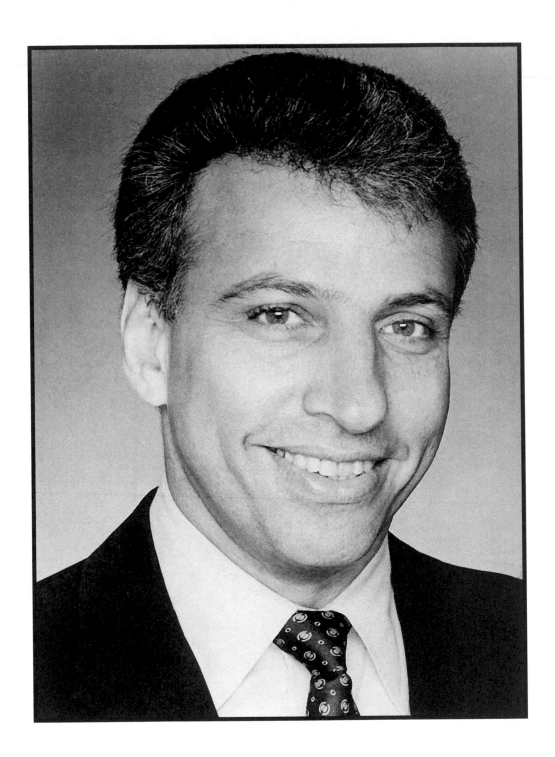

H. RONALD HULNICK
UNIVERSITY PRESIDENT

13 PSYCHIC SURGERY

BORN
June 5, 1939, Brooklyn, New York

EDUCATION
Ph.D., educational psychology and counseling, New Mexico State University

M.S., Clinical Psychology, Long Island University

CAREER HIGHLIGHTS
President, University of Santa Monica: 1983 to present

Co-authored with Dr. Mary R. Hulnick, *Financial Freedom in Eight Minutes a Day*: 1994

"I still have a hard time believing what took place. It continues to be one of the most amazing things that ever happened to me. And all these years later, it still doesn't make any sense."

H. Ronald Hulnick, Ph.D., president of the University of Santa Monica, exudes confidence, caution, and conservatism.

He is also about the last person you would expect to undergo psychic surgery, but a sudden seizure that left him bleeding and an old knee injury changed his mind.

Psychic surgery—or paranormal healing, as it is sometimes called—is a tough concept to accept. It challenges everything anybody ever learned in biology about how the body works, and few people with a science degree seem to give it much credence.

Psychic surgeons have no formal medical training. They conduct no tests, take no x rays, use no anesthesia. Yet within moments of diagnosing your problem, they will operate using nothing more than their hands or a knife that never seems to cause bleeding. They may never even touch you. Instead, they may simply hold their hands two or three inches above your body to effect their healing.

You're wide awake through the whole thing. And when it's all over, your "surgeon" proclaims you cured and you're able to walk out of the surgeon's office as if no operation had taken place. No intensive care. No week-long recovery. No forms to fill out.

In the United States, that scenario is almost impossible to believe. So how did Ron Hulnick get so lucky?

"I wish it was simply a case of intellectual curiosity that first led me to check out psychic surgery," says Ron. "But it began with a call from a close friend. She was on her way to Mexico to have psychic surgery performed. Being in her seventies, she wanted someone to accompany her on the trip, and even though I was skeptical about what she was getting into, I agreed to join her.

"My friend had been suffering from an uncomfortable condition that can cause extreme bloating. She contracted it as a young girl after coming down with rheumatic fever. Every six to eight months, in a medical procedure, she literally had her body pumped out to get rid of fluids. The liquids gathered everywhere: her legs, stomach, arms—you name it. She was always bloated."

The condition was difficult to live with and Ron's friend finally decided to zip over the border to rural Mexico to try psychic surgery.

"We arrived in the surgeon's office to find a waiting room filled with people the mainstream medical profession had either failed or given up on," says Ron. "You got the feeling they were in search of a miracle and willing to try anything."

That made Ron suspicious.

"You've got to remember that my conservative profession and training had not prepared me to deal with anything like this," says Ron. "I approached it like a scientist. To say that I was highly skeptical would be an understatement."

But Ron put his doubts aside long enough to help his friend. "I reasoned that since I had come this far, I might as well keep an open mind," says Ron.

A short while later Ron and his elderly friend were led into a tiny room where they were introduced to the psychic surgeon, simply called Feliciano.

"It wasn't a formal introduction," says Ron. "Feliciano spoke very little English, maybe a few words that he had picked up treating other Americans."

The surgeon began his work. "He seemed to know what her problem was without asking her any questions," Ron says. "But given her condition, I wasn't impressed."

Still, Ron remained by his friend's side. "Mainly he moved his hands around her body, like in a massage, touching her here and there. Nothing really seemed to be going on. And as I sat there I remained as skeptical as when I first walked through the door."

RON'S TURN ON THE TABLE

Sitting in the room observing his friend, Ron tried to maintain a professional skepticism, but all that was about to be dramatically altered. "Without any warning whatsoever, I became ill," says Ron. "I was nauseous, and I knew I needed a bathroom fast. I clutched my stomach and ran out of the room and down the hall to the nearest men's room."

Ron made it to the bathroom, then passed out cold. "I was having a seizure," Ron explains. "I came to a few moments later to find myself lying on the bathroom floor, blood dripping from my nose. I realized I'd blacked out and smashed my nose on the floor."

Hearing the thump of Ron's body hitting the bathroom floor, Feliciano's assistant ran in to find him lying on the cement. She summoned help and had him carried back to the treatment room.

"Groggy, I looked up to see the surgeon's assistant standing over me," recalls Ron. "I remember thinking, 'Oh great! Here I've come all this way to help my friend and before her treatment has ended, they're carrying her off the table to put me on it.'"

But Ron didn't ask the surgeon any questions. He knew he needed whatever help was around. "I wasn't strong enough to do much of anything, so I let Feliciano do his work," Ron says. "He gently put his hand on my face and nose and the bleeding stopped.

"When it was clear Feliciano was finished, I turned to get up from the table," recalls Ron. But before he could make it to the door, Feliciano called out: "You need work." Ron was tempted to keep on moving, but there was something in the way Feliciano called out that made him want to stay.

"It could have been the way he looked at me," says Ron. "It was as if he were seeing right through me into my mind. His gaze was piercing."

Ron found himself lying back down. "Feliciano put his hands behind my head and ran his fingers up and down the back of my skull. I had no idea what he was up to. Then Feliciano spoke again. 'You fall down as a child, hit your head. You have seizures. I fix.'

"I was speechless over the accuracy of what he had said," Ron recalls. "It was true. As a child I had taken a fall and hit the back of my head. I remembered that. It was also true that just about every seven years since that fall I had experienced convulsive seizures. But I had never thought to tie the two together."

In fact, it had been nearly seven years since Ron's last seizure. "I didn't have much time to think about the whole thing," says Ron. "It all went so fast. He worked on the back of my head. I have no idea what he was doing. I couldn't see, nor could I feel much of anything. It was like a gentle massage, his hands moving around, but I didn't know what he was doing.

"Feliciano did manage to stop the bleeding. But when it came to the seizures, I was looking for more proof than that to believe I was really through with them."

When Feliciano moved away from his head, Ron rose from the table to leave. "I thought I was finished, but my friend had a different idea," Ron says. "She suggested I stay and tell Feliciano about an old ski injury that had been plaguing my knee for years. On a fairly regular basis, my knee would pop out of place."

Years of experience had taught Ron how to pop the knee back into place. But it was painful and frustrating. Each episode would be followed by weeks of soreness. "Whenever my knee popped out, about all I wanted to do was stay in bed," says Ron. "In fact, I had just gotten over an episode prior to this trip."

The remembrance of his pain coupled with his friend's urging convinced Ron to allow Feliciano to treat his problem. "I sat back down," Ron says. This time, Ron sat in a chair. "I was close enough to see everything he was doing."

Yet what happened next was so completely bizarre, Ron didn't believe his own eyes.

"He put his hands on my knee and I saw my knee transformed from skin and bones to a thick liquid," Ron recalls. "Feliciano's hands then *entered* my knee and moved this liquid stuff around."

Was Ron hallucinating? Was he still groggy from his fall?

Shaking his head, Ron continued. "Sure I was shocked to see what he did to my knee, but I know I wasn't imagining it. It all happened before my eyes. His hand had literally entered my knee and dissolved my skin to liquid. I didn't feel a thing."

However surreal, Ron's tale has been told countless times by other patients who have undergone psychic surgery. Many report that the psychic surgeon removed lumps or diseased tissue from the liquid mass the surgeon had apparently created.

"Feliciano didn't pull anything out of my body, he simply ran his hands through this liquid stuff which was once my knee," Ron says. "Believe me, I know how hard this is to understand. I was there and I still have trouble. I still to this day can't believe what took place. The surgery took about twenty seconds. And when the surgeon removed his hand and my knee returned to normal, it was as if it had never happened.

"I kept saying, 'I must be dreaming.' But I wasn't. I had experienced it all. I had looked down and seen my own knee turn to liquid.

"At the end of our session, Feliciano did one final thing," adds Ron. "He picked up a Bible, pointed to a passage and instructed me to read. I don't remember what it was, but I think it was his way of sealing the session, a kind of postsurgery prescription to make sure that whatever had been cured would not recur."

Returning to his hotel room, Ron was stunned by what had taken place. "I spent the day in disbelief," he says. "Had it not been for a red spot that was left on my knee, I would have doubted anything had ever taken place. The spot lasted for about half the day. Then suddenly this tiredness came over me. Exhaustion. I just had to sleep.

"I stayed in bed for the next day and a half. I was really tired. The only explanation I could give for it was that my body needed time to regenerate itself—to incorporate the healing that had just taken place."

A MIND/BODY CONNECTION?

It's been fifteen years since Ron saw Feliciano. And although psychic surgery worked for him, his friend was not so fortunate. She continued to have problems related to swelling.

Why should one person be healed and another not? No one really knows.

Some psychic surgeons feel that while a patient's belief or disbelief can affect the success of psychic surgery, it is the postoperative beliefs that sometimes sabotage healing. It's impossible to verify—as are most claims related to psychic surgery—but some patients have felt that when they began to doubt that healing had taken place, their health problems returned.

Although firmly ingrained in the disciplines of Western science, Ron was nonetheless open to this type of thinking. "I have since come to a greater understanding of the connection between mind, body, and spirit, especially when it comes to health," he says. "As a psychologist and educator, I know the power of the mind and how it can affect healing. And over the years now I've had many patients and students who [have] used their minds to successfully alter and improve their health."

That's why "I've worked to stay as aware as I possibly can about how my mind, emotions, and spiritual beliefs impact my overall health."

But has psychic surgery actually converted Ron into a bona fide psychic surgery "believer"?

"I don't know about labeling me a 'believer,'" he says honestly. "All I can say is that it's been fifteen years since my treatment in Mexico. And given that

I haven't had a seizure or knee problem since, psychic surgery definitely worked for me."

SPOTLIGHT ON PSYCHIC SURGERY

Diagnosing without checking symptoms? Operating without a scalpel or a laser? No anesthesia necessary? If that sounds reasonable to you, then welcome to the world of psychic surgery.

Experts who have looked into this therapy report that a psychic surgeon usually feels he has the ability to diagnose without benefit of standard medical testing, even if there are no physical signs of the disease or ailment present. And although psychic surgeons may never have seen the inside of a real laboratory or science classroom, most claim they have an inherent understanding of how the body works and how it can be healed.

Where do they get their knowledge? Many claim that it comes from God. And they seem to see themselves as corporeal entities through which God performs medical treatment. They conduct "operations" that purportedly remove everything from tumors to AIDS, and they operate on unsedated patients who instantly heal without a scar.

It should not be surprising that much of this type of surgery takes place in small, rural villages on makeshift tables and chairs. Nor should it be surprising that 95 percent of all surgeries involve little more than the laying on of hands to remove "bad blood" from the body.

Just where and when this alternative healing practice originated is hard to figure out. In the Philippines they are able to trace it back to 1521, when European adventurers first came in contact with the native peoples of these islands and witnessed firsthand this kind of healing work. Some historians believe that there was a small region of this island nation from which hundreds of healers came and whose ancestors still practice today.

Today in the Philippines—and Mexico as well—psychic surgeons are as common as family physicians are in the United States. And in Great Britain, psychic surgeons have been allowed to treat patients in 1,500 national hospitals located throughout the country—although it is accurate to say they are simply tolerated. Allowed to perform their "miracles," they are not permitted compensation other than transportation costs.

There are claims that several million people throughout the world are treated by psychic surgeons every year. In Brazil, for example, the famous healer Arigo was said to have healed hundreds of people a day. In fact, his reputation for a quick surgical fix was so widespread that upon his death, the October 16, 1972, issue of *Time* reported, "he claimed to be guided by the wise voice of a long-deceased physician who he had never known personally. The uneducated healer saw as many as 300 patients a day, diagnosing and treating them in minutes. He treated almost every known ailment, and most of his patients not only survived but actually improved or recovered."

Whatever the physical condition, there seems to be a psychic surgeon practicing in that specialty. While medical doctors often warn that psychic surgery is a con game practiced on desperately ill people, advocates of this therapy believe that true healing can occur. They believe that most successful surgery starts with the patient's belief that they can be cured, that the body is capable of healing itself, and that the psychic surgeon is a tool through which a greater power makes this healing possible.

Still interested? Take the time to research your psychic healer thoroughly. Referrals by people who have actually worked with the practitioner are a good place to start. While many healers seem to have a genuine gift, a few have been proven to be charlatans. And you probably won't find your practitioner just around the corner either. You may need to travel outside the United States to find a surgeon, who may live in a remote location where the only directions you'll receive are to "turn right at the end of the village." And forget about health insurance, receptionists, or even getting an appointment. In these remote spots, you show up and take your chances.

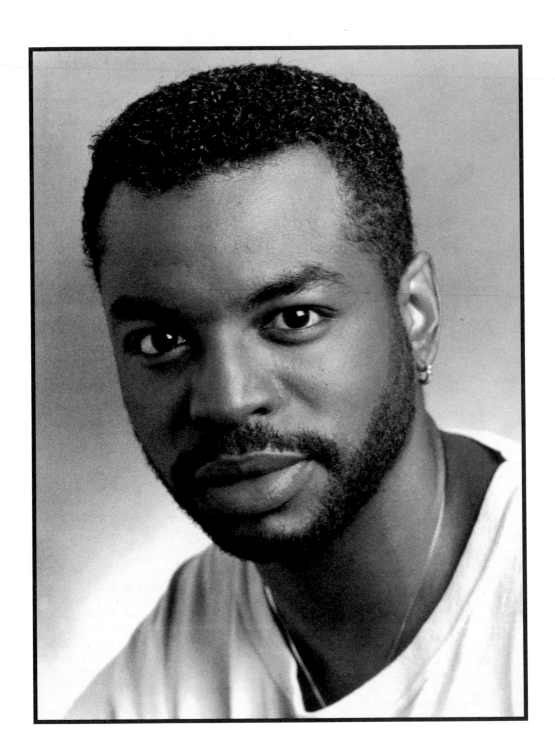

14 ROLFING

BORN
1957, Landstuhl, Germany

EDUCATION
B.F.A., University of Southern
California

CAREER HIGHLIGHTS
FILM
Looking for Mr. Goodbar
The Hunter
Star Trek Generations
Star Trek Voyager

TELEVISION
"Roots"
"Star Trek: The Next Generation"
"A Roots Christmas:
Kunta Kinte's Gift"
"Christy"
"Dummy"
"Once in a Million:
The Ron LeFlore Story"
"Reading Rainbow"
(host and co-producer)

"Rolfing can be a very dramatic, very freeing experience."

Twenty years ago, LeVar Burton, the beloved star of "Reading Rainbow," "Roots," and "Star Trek: The Next Generation," was a serious seminary student intent on the priesthood.

Today he is a major player in the development of new films and other entertainment media at Peaceful Warrior Productions, the company he launched in California's San Fernando Valley.

Yet the distance LeVar has traveled from priesthood to producer is shorter than one might imagine. Because although LeVar has changed vocations, he has not changed his life's focus. He is still committed to his faith, spiritual exploration, and God—which is why Peaceful Warrior Productions is one of those rare businesses with a cloth-covered altar set up in the office of its chief executive officer.

"I see my work in this world as an absolutely sacred journey," explains LeVar as he lights a candle and places it carefully on his office altar. "I try to remind myself of the sacred nature of this existence whenever and wherever I can. So I use the altar to remind myself that there is a focus of spirit in all I do."

It's not something LeVar has always been able to do.

By his own account, LeVar was a very different person when he shot to stardom at age nineteen in the television miniseries "Roots." The series held the nation enthralled for almost a week as it revealed centuries of rich African-American history and culture. But by the end of the first night's viewing, a young African slave by the name of Kunta Kinte held the country by its heartstrings. LeVar Burton had come to symbolize the innocence, goodness, and natural beauty found in all primitive societies. " 'Roots' was my first thing as an actor," says LeVar. "It aired for eight consecutive nights, but my part was over in two. So in one weekend, I went from oblivion to stardom."

Unfortunately, post-"Roots" fame was overwhelming for a young boy who grew up on an American military base in Germany. "My ego got way out control," admits LeVar, "and it caused a major crisis in my life. It was an experience that really shook me."

It was also the major reason why LeVar fell in and out of relationships for the year after his success on "Roots." He couldn't seem to give or get what he wanted in any relationship. And every time he started to get really close to someone, he managed to sabotage the relationship—even with the one woman who loved him deeply.

LeVar declines to reveal any details, but he says, "When I blew it with this woman, I knew I needed to take a long hard look at myself, at what I wanted, and what I was getting. I knew I needed help. I knew I needed to make some serious and dramatic changes in both my behavior and in how I felt about myself.

"That's when I made a pledge that, whatever it took, I would dedicate myself to achieving balance in my life—emotionally, mentally, physically, and especially spiritually.

"I had no idea what I was going to do," adds the actor. "But I knew I needed to open up in order to grow. I recognized that traditional psychotherapy seemed like a good place to start, but because I wanted to bring all of me into alignment—both physically and emotionally—I realized that therapy alone was not going to be enough. I wanted to go at this balance thing, this wholeness thing, no holds barred.

"I wanted to just jump in."

THE HEALING PATH

LeVar tried a number of alternative healing therapies. But it wasn't until a year after losing the woman who adored him that he found the right combination of therapies to help him achieve balance.

LeVar used psychotherapy to open himself up emotionally, and Rolfing, a ten-session intensive bodywork therapy, to physically release the long-held tensions that plagued his body.

LeVar believed that past physical and emotional trauma had created both physical and emotional rigidity. This resulted in tightened muscles and destructive relationships. His body and mind were out of alignment, which is why LeVar felt such a need for balance in his life—and probably why his back hurt and his hip muscles always felt tight.

LeVar was born with flat feet, which contributed to his lower back pain. The goal of LeVar's Rolfer was to create arches in LeVar's feet where none existed before and to loosen up LeVar's tightened muscles by applying pressure with his fingers, elbows, and knuckles. This would stretch the thin fascial membrane that encases the muscles. Rolfers explain that, over a period of years, muscle tightness causes the fascia to contract. Then, the body subtly contorts itself to accommodate the contraction. Rolfers attempt to stretch the fascia back out to allow the muscles to flex and return to their natural position. The entire body will then be realigned to work with the earth's gravitational forces. It will be "balanced."

Rolfing also provides emotional benefits. As the body is freed from physical blockage and stress, emotional traumas seem to be released. Inventor Ida Rolf, Ph.D., reports in her book *Ida Rolf Talks About Rolfing*: "Rolfing is not primarily a psychotherapeutic approach to the problems of humans, but the effect it has had on the human psyche has been so noteworthy that many people insist on so regarding it. Rolfing is an approach to the personality through the myofascial collagen components of the physical body. It integrates and balances the so-called other bodies of man . . . The psychological, emotional, mental, and spiritual aspects."

Anticipating some of these benefits, LeVar went to his first Rolfing session. "The office was very warm, with incense burning, soft music in the background, and a nice fire burning in the fireplace," says LeVar.

"Before lying down on the treatment table, the Rolfer and I discussed my personal history and my goals. Physically, I was having some lower back pain, my hips were tight, and I wanted my spine to get a little straighter. Psychologically, by identifying and processing any emotional blocks, I was hoping that they would no longer be able to affect me as an adult. At that point, I was in therapy twice a week so I was really getting to the core of a lot of emotional issues."

LeVar and the Rolfer worked together for ten sessions over a twenty-week period. Each session lasted around sixty to ninety minutes, with the Rolfer kneading and pressing on every muscle in LeVar's body. Eventually the therapist broke through the physical rigidity that had entrapped the actor for close to thirty years.

There were psychological breakthroughs too. "Going into that office every week, I never knew what I was going to talk about," says LeVar. Sometimes he talked about issues that had arisen in ongoing psychotherapy sessions; other times it seemed that long-forgotten memories would suddenly emerge.

"There was a very specific childhood trauma I had blocked out," says LeVar. "I am not willing to talk about it. But in order to protect myself, so that I might continue to operate in everyday life, I shut down the part of myself that had contact with that experience. I didn't even remember it until almost twenty-five years later, as I was being Rolfed.

"When I did remember, it gave me a piece of my own puzzle that made absolute sense. All of a sudden, I could see in this one piece of information—'Oh my God! That's why I have this or that issue in my life. That's where it comes from!' "

The idea that memories could be stored away was a concept that LeVar easily accepted. "Let me tell you about an experience I had during the shooting of 'Roots,'" offers the actor. "Alex Haley had given me an early copy of his book and had me read sections of it. Then we went into a warehouse down in Savannah where the hull of the ship had been re-created. We shot for three consecutive days. I remember vaguely going in on the beginning of the first day, and that was the last thing I remembered.

"What happened to me during the course of the re-creation of those scenes was that some genetic sense memory took over, and I relived that incident from a place inside of me that had lived the experience before.

"I had no concept of time, getting up in the morning, taking a shower, or going to the set. I don't remember those three days clearly. I just have vague images and shadows."

Perhaps because LeVar easily accepted the recall of forgotten memories, he was able to release through Rolfing the emotional rigidity that had created his difficulties in relationships. "The more time I spent on the table, the more I began to realize that I could go to the places where those memories were stored—the places I wanted to run away from. I could take my awareness there, then breathe into that place and release its pain."

But equally powerful was the self-knowledge LeVar gained as he reexamined the beliefs he held about himself.

"Sometimes the Rolfer would be working and a belief I held about myself would come up," explains LeVar. "So during the session, I would examine that belief to see if it was true. One time, the Rolfer was working one part of my body and I became overwhelmed with a sense of being unworthy, of not feeling 'good enough' in my life. And I realized that, despite the success I had attained, I had walked around for more than twenty years of my life feeling like I wasn't enough. You know that feeling: 'Everyone else is better—I have to do more to be accepted, get better grades, perform better than they did.'

"That belief wasn't serving me at all. But it was brought to my attention through Rolfing so I could then deal with it in a conscious way. I could say to myself, 'That's no longer true. That's a lie.'"

Being able to let go of his feelings of inadequacy and see himself in a new way left LeVar overcome with emotion and with a newfound sense of personal power.

"I always felt great after each of the sessions," says the actor. "I wanted to eat. I was famished. I was really solid and I finally felt totally at home in my body."

On a physical level, LeVar's spine had become straighter, which eased the pain he had been experiencing in his lower back. And on an emotional level, LeVar had finally achieved the balance he had sought. He was finally able to establish a stable, loving relationship with the beautiful woman who is now his wife and the mother of his child.

"Who I am today is the sum total of all my experience," says LeVar.

SPOTLIGHT ON ROLFING

Although it may seem odd to actually pay someone to dig into your body with their knuckles and elbows or poke you with their fingers, that's exactly what happens when you sign up for a course of Rolfing, a bodywork technique developed by the late chemist Ida Rolf, Ph.D.

Rolfing was designed to improve posture and eliminate chronic pain and tightened muscles by firmly kneading, poking, and prodding muscles to stretch out the thin fascial membrane that encases them. In some cases, it has also helped its adherents release the emotional pain of old traumas locked inside their minds and bodies. The result, Rolfers say, is a reintegration of mind and body so that both are balanced, along with a physical realignment with the earth's gravitational pull.

By all accounts, Ida Rolf first became interested in bodywork when an osteopath fixed a breathing problem she had developed after being kicked by a horse. From that point on, Dr. Rolf was convinced that a person's physiological health could be improved by realigning the overall structure of the body. Combining her knowledge of yoga with the structural realignment of osteopathic manipulation, she designed a form of bodywork called structural integration—affectionately nicknamed "Rolfing" by its practitioners.

Eventually Dr. Rolf founded the Rolf Institute for Structural Integration in Boulder, Colorado, a training school that today boasts more than 800 graduate Rolfers.

Rolfing was popular during the seventies, but by the early eighties it had developed a reputation for being painful. People had begun to turn away from it. In response, Rolfers developed gentler techniques to achieve the same results. Today, Rolfing has found an enthusiastic new audience.

Rolfing works to counteract the years that most of us spend slumping in chairs, leaning against walls and standing in supermarket checkouts—all of which throw our bodies out of alignment. And to make matters worse, as one part of the body goes out of line, other parts try to compensate. That, Rolfers say, causes muscles to contract in unnatural ways. After years of this type of contracture, the fascial membrane covering the muscles shrinks as well, restricting the free movement of joints and muscles.

"The problem can be further aggravated by accidents, injuries, and stress," says Scot Spann, former director of the Rolfing Institute. In fact, stress throws the body out of alignment just as surely as if it had been thrown against a wall. The body will compensate just as if it had been physically injured. It will develop protective postures—hunched shoulders, for example, which negatively affect posture and body balance.

Our occupations also can aggravate our bodies, particularly if we're forced to perform repetitive motions. Assembly line workers, meat cutters, or carpenters who may use one side of their body more than the other, simply because they're left- or right-handed, often benefit from Rolfing.

The Rolfer uses hands, arms, and elbows to apply deep pressure to the contracted area in an effort to release the constricted fascia. This is done systematically, from head to toe, in ten sessions over ten weeks, until the entire body has been worked.

At the beginning of the Rolfing process, both Rolfer and client review the client's goals. A photo is taken of the patient standing to show how and where the body is out of alignment. The actual work is done with the client lying prone on a massage table.

In the first three sessions, the Rolfer works on the outer fascia, loosening up superficial, or recently acquired, stresses. The next three sessions work on fundamental patterns that were often established in the person's formative years. The seventh session works with the head. The goal of this session is to align the head with the neck and shoulders so that the head can now rest in its natural relationship to the rest of the body. The last three sessions integrate all of the previous work.

After the initial ten-session series, people are usually advised to come in for a tune-up every year or so, or whenever some extreme physical or emotional trauma may affect the alignment.

Rolfing is most effective in eliminating chronic back pain, structural or postural problems, curvatures of the spine, and minor aches and pains. As the body is balanced, respiratory problems are often cleared and people report a greater breathing capacity, which is why Rolfing is particularly appreciated by singers and entertainers.

Once aligned and reintegrated, the physical body improves, often dramatically. Dental problems such as temporomandibular joint syndrome are relieved, headaches disappear, and people report feeling lighter on their feet, more graceful. Dancers say they are better able to execute more difficult dance patterns, while athletes report greater physical endurance and improvement in their playing, as their true center of gravity has been restored. Perhaps that's why some baseball players for the San Francisco Giants, the New York Mets, the Los Angeles Dodgers, and the New York Yankees have been Rolfed—including former Mets pitcher Craig Swan, who believes that if he had been Rolfed early in his career, he'd still be pitching.

But this is only one side of the Rolfing story. Although Ida Rolf originally designed Structural Integration to treat physical problems, the Rolf Institute reports that one out of every four people now uses Rolfing to treat psychological problems. When the therapy is used in this way, the body is seen as a gateway to the mind and emotions.

No one is sure why or how this works, but as Rolfing releases old hurts, people report that depression lifts, sleep improves, and decision-making comes more easily. They no longer feel weighed down by lingering memories, and they say they are emotionally healthier and happier.

If you want to get started before your first appointment, however, stand in front of a mirror and review your posture and stance. Then, stretch your hands up over your head and return them to the side of your body. Doesn't that simple stretching make your whole body feel better? Start noticing the way you walk, the posture you take while sitting in front of your computer, or while standing as you cook. Can it be improved?

Of course. And Rolfing is one way to do it.

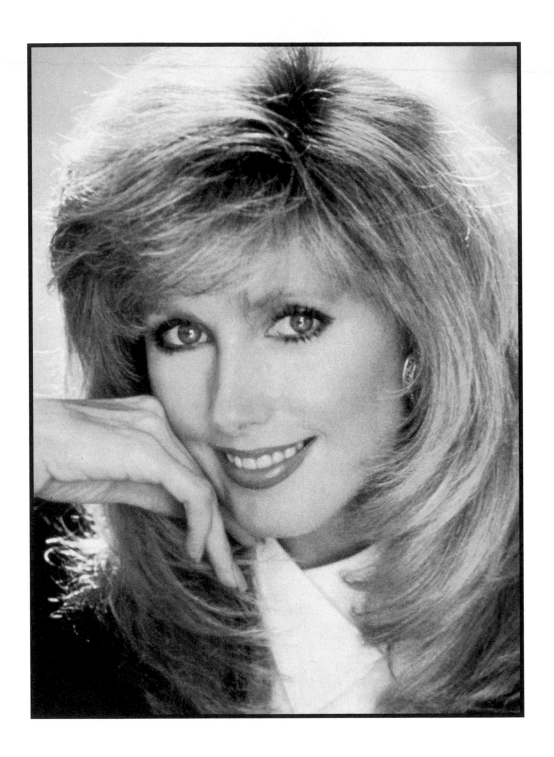

MORGAN FAIRCHILD
ACTRESS

15 TRADITIONAL CHINESE HERBAL MEDICINE

"I knew that Chinese herbal medicine wouldn't be a panacea that worked overnight. I never expected instant relief...With what I was going through, I knew I needed to bolster my immune system and that would take time."

BORN
Dallas, Texas

PROFESSIONAL AWARDS
Golden Globe nomination, 1982:
"Flamingo Road"
Emmy nomination, 1990:
"Murphy Brown"

CAREER HIGHLIGHTS
TELEVISION
"Falcon Crest"
"Paper Dolls"
"Roseanne"
"The Memory of Eva Ryker"
"The Initiation of Sarah"
"North & South"
"The Haunting of Sarah Hardy"

FILM
The Seduction
Midnight Cop

THEATER
Geniuses
Goodbye, Charlie

BOOKS
Super Looks

Morgan Fairchild was exhausted. The exquisitely delicate actress with her magnificent mane of blond hair could hardly get out of bed. True, she did work fourteen-hour days sandwiched between workouts, star-studded outings and nurturing an eight-year relationship. But that never used to faze her. She thrived on activity. Yet now, no matter how much rest or sleep she got, she never, ever, felt truly rested.

What was going on?

Morgan went to see an ear, nose, and throat doctor, who believed her fatigue was the result of the Epstein-Barr virus, and that she had chronic fatigue syndrome. Morgan was caught off guard. "I had just read about the virus and didn't recognize any symptoms," she says.

But her doctor persisted. "He asked if I had been tired and I told him, 'Sure I'm tired.' After all, I had just finished shooting a TV movie where we worked both days and nights. Everybody on the set was ready to drop."

The doctor sent Morgan for blood tests. "The test results showed that I had elevated Epstein-Barr antibodies," she reports. That's not uncommon, but combined with Morgan's continuing lethargy and a previous diagnosis of Candida, a yeastlike infection that is sometimes seen as a symptom of chronic fatigue, her doctor suspected she might have the beginnings of chronic fatigue syndrome. As time went on, she developed memory loss, bloating, and depression—all classic symptoms of the problem.

"I was up a whole dress size," Morgan says. "My face looked like a pumpkin, and I was living in sweaters and leggings because nothing fit.

"I tried not eating to get rid of the bloating. But I was starving myself and still gaining weight. It's very discouraging when nothing you do seems to do any good. It's especially hard when you have never had a weight problem."

Morgan was dismayed to learn that when it came to a cure, conventional medicine could do little for chronic fatigue syndrome. But Morgan is a strong person. And like most people with a chronic infection, she found her own way to deal with the overwhelming fatigue: She gave up her social life. "I saved whatever energy I had for work," says the actress. "Each day on the set was an uphill battle. I had a lot of problems with my memory. I went from having a steel-trap mind to suddenly not being able to recall phone numbers that I'd known for years."

And while a supportive relationship remained intact throughout her ordeal, Morgan was forced to give up another love—the gym.

"Even when I'm on location, I try to work out five or six days a week," Morgan says. "But I had to cut back dramatically. At first I tried to work right through the illness, and then I realized all it did was make things worse. I just had to quit."

But Morgan wouldn't quit searching for a cure. "I read all the books and tried to do what they said," says the actress. "I even went on a very restrictive diet, eating nothing but brown rice, steamed vegetables and a little chicken for protein, but it didn't help."

Morgan tried to tough it out, but, "at some point you just start wondering where you're going," she says. "It gets very depressing because you really don't know what to do."

But fate wasn't about to let her down. A rare night out for the now semi-reclusive actress found her dining at Spago. Morgan, formerly a steady customer of the trendy eatery, was greeted effusively by her friend Bernard, the maître d'.

Previously, Bernard had revealed to Morgan that he had the same health problems she did. "But that night he was looking very svelte and dapper—no longer bloated like he'd been. I said to him, 'Oh my God, what have you done?' He told me about a doctor of Oriental medicine he was seeing in Beverly Hills and how the doctor had had a lot of success treating patients like me."

Wasting no time, Morgan called the doctor's office for an appointment. But Mark Holmes, O.M.D., couldn't see her until Christmas Eve, a few days away. And, to make matters worse, Morgan came down with what she believed was the flu.

When Morgan arrived for her first appointment, the doctor began his investigation by applying the four principles of diagnosis in Chinese herbal medicine: *observation,* looking over the patient's overall complexion, facial color, skin tone, fingernails, and tongue; *interrogation,* asking the patient about any symptoms like night sweats, chills, or coughing; *auscultation,* listening to the sounds of the organs as he gently "knocks" on the stomach, back, and extremities; and *palpation,* feeling the pulses located on both wrists, the head and neck area, and acupuncture points on the head, neck, arms, and upper back.

"Once Dr. Holmes finished his examination, he told me, 'You don't have the flu, you have a bacterial sinus infection and need to be on antibiotics.'" It was not exactly what she was expecting to hear from a doctor of Oriental medicine, but Dr. Holmes recognized Morgan's infection needed antibiotics. He also confirmed the diagnosis of Morgan's ear, nose, and throat specialist: She was, indeed, suffering from chronic fatigue syndrome. He could help fight the chronic fatigue, Dr. Holmes assured his patient, but it really wouldn't be that effective until the sinus infection was taken care of.

"He sent me right over to my ear, nose, and throat doctor to get a prescription," says Morgan. But before she left, Morgan was given an acupuncture treatment in which Dr. Holmes stuck needles in her hands and legs at acupuncture points that he felt would help fight her sinus infection. She was also given several Chinese herbs: *pe min kan wan*, an herb in pill form to fight her sinus infection, and two herbal mixtures—*ginseng* and *astragalus* to boost her immune system, and *ginseng* and *atractylodes* to eliminate her persistent abdominal bloating.

Dr. Holmes also suspected that there was an emotional problem plaguing Morgan. In Chinese medicine, the outer body is seen as representative of the inner consciousness. Therefore, before a patient can be successfully treated, inner issues must be addressed.

"He spotted right away that I was having problems with a family member," Morgan recalls. "It was then that I realized that the relationship was affecting my body and inhibiting my ability to respond to treatment. Stress of any kind with an Epstein-Barr infection is very difficult. And the more I learn about stress the more I believe that emotional stress of any kind really wrecks your immune system."

A SLOW RECOVERY

That year, instead of flying home to her family in Dallas for Christmas, Morgan spent Christmas Day in bed with a horrible headache. "But at least I had the antibiotics and herbs and took comfort in knowing I was on my way to getting well," says the actress.

The following week, Morgan returned to Dr. Holmes. "He gave me more herbs, which I took three or four times a day. I made sure to keep them with me at all times." The herbs were *hsiao yao wan* to aid her liver, which Dr. Holmes felt had been affected by the virus. Dr. Holmes also did more acupuncture, this time focusing on points on her feet, which are thought to help release toxins the body might be harboring.

"I knew that Chinese herbal medicine wouldn't be a panacea that worked overnight," Morgan says. "I never expected instant relief. As Americans we get very spoiled because we're used to antibiotics or things where you take a pill and it works and you're instantly cured. But with what I was going through I knew I needed to bolster my immune system and that it would take time."

Little by little Morgan began to see signs she was returning to her old self. "I started having days where I actually woke up and felt like doing things like going to lunch with friends," recalls the actress. "I remember being at this little shopping center that I go to and having one of the saleswomen say to me, 'Oh, we were just talking about you.' It seems one of their customers had seen me and couldn't believe I was running around without makeup. The customer thought it made me look really bad. The saleswoman defended me, saying that she thought I looked pretty with or without makeup.

"I said, 'Oh honey, you don't have to defend me. I feel so lucky feeling well enough to be shopping that I don't care if anybody thinks I look good or bad. All that matters is that I got out of the house today!'"

RIDING THE ROLLER COASTER

Knowing that she was on the road to recovery made Morgan's slow healing more bearable.

"My health went up and down for a long while, but I learned how to deal with it," Morgan says. "I exercised on days I felt I could and [on] other days, I just didn't. I had good periods, but if I worked too hard, I found myself sliding right back down from stress. As time went on, I was able to handle more and more stress before sliding back. So I went backward and forward for a while before I was fully back on my feet."

By spring, Morgan was remembering phone numbers, working out, and fitting into her clothes. "My body never returned to where it was before the illness," says Morgan, "because it all happened at an age when everything starts to fall. So no matter how many visits I make to the gym, I'm still paying for my illness."

But don't waste your time worrying about how Morgan is taking this. These days all she really cares about is how to reduce the stress in her life, knowing it could sabotage her immune system and cause a relapse. "I found one really good technique," laughs Morgan. "You learn to say no. You stop caring if people will like you because you have to say no. In my position, I'm always pressured to do something—to go here and give a speech or come to dinner because so-and-so really wants to meet you or they really need this photo session or interview and it would mean so much. But I have learned to say no.

"I also learned to establish parameters. Sometimes even things I really love to do I can't. I used to go jetting around the country to places like Washington, giving speeches twice a week. Now, I accept the fact that maybe I could do that once a month."

Morgan also tries to see Dr. Holmes every week or two. Her chronic infections may be a thing of the past, but she still gets the occasional stomach virus or cold, just like the rest of us. "My treatments are now preventive, trying to head things off at the pass," says Morgan. "I've had a lot fewer sinus infections than before. If I feel something's coming on, my doctor will either prescribe something or do acupuncture.

"I try to stay away from antibiotics, which, in me, tend to bring on candidiasis. I know that my body is prone to such infections. But one of the things I immediately liked about Dr. Holmes was that he was not afraid to recommend things like antibiotics when they are the only thing that could help. But with the maintenance program I'm on, I need so much less."

Morgan also likes the fact that she and Dr. Holmes are partners in her health care. "He doesn't do it *for* me," Morgan says. "Even with the herbs, I still have to get my rest, pace myself, learn how to deal with stress, take the herb pills he gives me, and be sensitive to my body and its health. If I don't feel like going out to dinner or a movie, I don't go. Listening to your body is so much of what Chinese herbal medicine is all about."

This doesn't mean Morgan is sitting home knitting afghans—not with movie roles taking her on location to Germany and Bosnia.

"In Berlin it was freezing and raining and snowing," remembers Morgan. "And while many others working on the film got sick, I never did. I kept on taking my herbs, as well as some herbal drops to help deal with jet lag. It all worked just great.

"I also made a movie in Bosnia that turned out to be a very stress-filled experience. There was lots of trouble on the set, but I stayed healthy. I even took time to explore. When the other actors went off to the casinos at night, I tagged along with the war correspondents to see what was really going on in these war-torn cities. I wanted to experience what I couldn't learn from *Time* or *Newsweek*."

Fortunately, Morgan made it back to Hollywood intact, and today she can often be found at Eclipse, a chic Hollywood restaurant owned by none other than Bernard, the former maître d' at Spago. But if you're lucky enough to be within earshot of Morgan and Bernard, don't expect to hear them dishing the latest Hollywood gossip. "When we get together the conversation always turns to our favorite health practitioner and Chinese herbal medicine," Morgan says. "After all, I don't think Bernard would have had the energy to open one of the most popular restaurants in town if he hadn't gotten help.

"Chinese herbal medicine has really made such a big difference in both our lives."

SPOTLIGHT ON TRADITIONAL CHINESE HERBAL MEDICINE

Do you have an "imbalance" in your "vital force"? Is your arthritis pain caused by "yang" suppressing "yin"?

Don't be too quick to answer unless you've already consulted a Chinese herbal medicine specialist. Although less familiar to westerners, these concepts have withstood the test of time throughout the Eastern hemisphere. For well over 3,000 years, Chinese herbal medicine specialists—considered analogous to mainstream physicians in China and other Asian countries—have been treating patients and bringing their bodies into "a state of harmony" or "balance," relieving their patients' pain and restoring their health.

But although this form of alternative health care dates back centuries, given the differences in diagnostic techniques, treatment, and even how the body is conceptualized, it may take another 3,000 years for the Western mind to fully understand it.

To develop that understanding, start by thinking of the body not as a unique machine that exists on its own but as a reflection of nature. The Chinese have spent thousands of years observing nature to explain how the body works. From these observations, they have formulated the Five Phase Theory, which suggests that each of nature's five elements—fire, earth, metal, water, and wood—have corresponding organs and functions within the human body.

Classically trained Chinese physicians explain disease as a breakdown of the delicate natural balance among these elements. So the goal of Chinese medicine is to balance elements and organs by bringing them back into harmony. To do that, they manipulate "yin" and "yang," terms that are simply used to reflect the complementary forces within any organism.

Continuing their analogy to nature, Chinese herbal medicine physicians speak in terms of the flow of energy and bodily fluids as they relate to the flow of the river and other waterways. When that energy—*qi* or *chi* (pronounced "chee"), or "vital life force," is blocked like a river unable to freely flow, the body is imbalanced and disease occurs. It is the job of the Chinese physician to unblock and release the energy, thus restoring the body's balance and health.

Just how do they do it? Forget exploratory procedures or x rays. These specialists generally rely on their own skills of observation, questioning, listening, smelling, and palpation to diagnose imbalances.

They'll begin by inspecting your face, tongue, hair, and complexion. They'll ask for medical complaints and wonder if you're cold or hot, how you feel when you wake up, or if you have any pain. They'll question you about your diet, interpersonal relationships, and general medical history. All the while they'll be listening to how you sound and smelling your body odor and breath. They may even ask for a sample of urine to smell and examine. Finally, they'll feel your pulse at both your wrists, stomach, and several key palpation points.

Pulse diagnosis is particularly important, practitioners agree. The specialist is checking the strength of your life energy. It's something like taking your blood pressure, and it is supposed to tell the specialist something about your internal organs.

Don't be surprised when your modern-day Chinese physician sends you off to the lab for a blood workup to confirm the diagnosis. Many doctors of Oriental medicine now incorporate the best of modern medicine to their arsenal of ancient techniques, recognizing the value of using both.

Regardless of how it is diagnosed, once your imbalance has been identified and the cause determined, a Chinese herbal medicine specialist will work to restore balance through a number of techniques.

The most common treatment in Chinese herbal medicine is herbs, generally in combinations of two or more. In fact, it is this practice of combining herbs—sometimes as many as nineteen—that has prevented Western scientists from studying or endorsing most herbal mixtures. Scientists can document the effects of one particular herb taken at one particular dose in one particular form and stored in one particular way. But figuring out not only how one herb works, but how it works when combined with the effects of other herbs, is not easy. It's complicated even more by the fact that each manufacturer processes and packages the herbs in a different way, and any of this handling can affect the strength and effectiveness of an herb. This is why more and more doctors of Oriental medicine are opting for pharmaceutical grades of herbs, which are sometimes available, but often at a higher cost.

Your best bet is to check that whoever is dispensing the herbs to you is state licensed or nationally certified in herbology. Many practitioners of herbology will actually grind their own herb mixtures in their office and give them to the patient in a packet to take before meals, a tea to be brewed, or a capsule to be taken several times a day. Regardless of who prepares them or where they come from, the best test is always how effective the herb is in curing whatever is ailing you.

Chinese physicians sometimes use massage to rebalance energy in the body, as well as acupuncture, an ancient practice that uses hair-thin, disposable needles inserted in critical points around the body to redirect the flow of energy. (See "Erie Mills—Acupuncture" on p. 1.)

As helpful as these treatments may be, Chinese medical specialists feel they have an equal obligation to prevent and cure disease. That's why a great deal of time is spent educating patients on how to take care of themselves. That's also why listening in on a consultation may sound a lot more like a poetry reading than a doctor's visit—especially when you hear the patient being told to "think of your body as a tree that needs to be dormant in the winter, growing in the spring, bearing fruit and maturing in summer, and shedding leaves in the fall."

Simply put, Chinese herbal medicine specialists teach that to achieve maximum health, you must follow the natural rhythms of nature.

Nature dictates that the summer and spring are times of activity and that fall and winter are times of rest. Each organ also has its own corresponding season and with the start of each season, a Chinese herbal medicine practitioner will pay extra attention to the corresponding organ. Fall signals the cooling down of the pulses and a time for less activity and more rest, while summer is naturally a time for less sleep, more activity, and a more active pulse. When these natural rhythms are followed, health ensues. When they're not, illness follows.

"People often become ill around Christmas because instead of following the natural flow which dictates extra rest in the winter, they wear themselves out shopping, going to parties, and with family activities," says Beverly Hills practitioner Mark Holmes, O.M.D.

What is our greatest stumbling block to living in the flow of nature? Living in large cities that tend to obliterate the natural, healing rhythms of human beings.

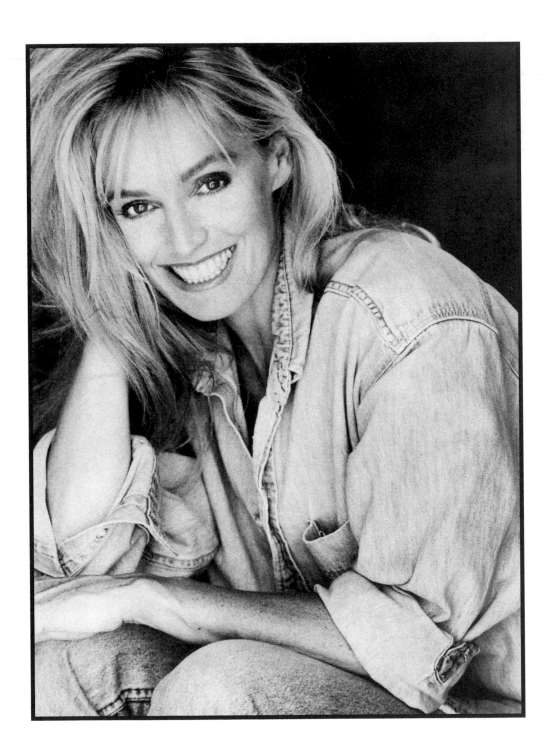

SUSAN ANTON
ACTRESS

BORN
October 12, 1950,
Yucaipa, California

PROFESSIONAL AWARDS
1992 & 1993 Honorary National
Crusade Chairperson of the
American Cancer Society

CAREER HIGHLIGHTS
U.S. Tour—Great Radio City
Music Hall Spectacular
with The Rockettes
Star Performer—
Las Vegas Flamingo

FILM
Goldengirl
Spring Fever
Cannonball Run

TELEVISION
"Baywatch"
"Presenting Susan Anton"
"Civil War"
"Quantum Leap"
"Night Court"

THEATER
Hurleyburley
The Will Rogers Follies

16 TRANSFORMATIONAL THERAPY

"Transformational therapy is a lot like preventive medicine—it helps keep our eyes open and located on our inner truths."

Before she discovered transformational therapy four years ago, Susan Anton was ready to give up on love—at least the kind that leads to marriage.

At age forty, the leggy, blond-haired talent had had her share of meaningful relationships, along with a good amount of professional success. But a failed marriage to a man whom she had trusted to be her husband and manager had left her believing that "living happily ever after" was indeed a fairy tale fed to little girls. She was seeing a guy, but she didn't consider him marriage material. And she was working, but not up to her potential.

The problem? "I'd lost passion," Susan admits. "I'd lost interest and I wasn't willing to put myself at risk anywhere. I was just treading water. I was playing this very conservative 'no risk—no gain' game with my life."

Of course, there were reasons, including Susan's failed marriage and a few significant relationships that had fizzled—Dudley Moore and Sylvester Stallone were two.

Then one day while working out at a gym on the Paramount Studios lot, she ran into her friend, fellow actor Leslie-Ann Warren. Leslie-Ann looked terrific, as usual. But as they talked, Susan realized that Leslie-Ann also appeared happier than she'd ever seen her. Susan asked Leslie-Ann what had transformed her into such a radiant person. Leslie-Ann told her about Breck Costin, a personal development specialist who ran transformational seminars covering everything from career to courtship.

In Costin's brand of transformational therapy, he works with individuals to help them identify and eliminate potentially limiting patterns so that they can experience greater personal freedom and move forward in life on personal and professional levels.

The basis of the seminars is the facilitator's ability to coach participants through any situations in which they need assistance—career, health, relationship issues—so that the clients are better able to understand and accept who they are, where they want to be, and what work is necessary to get there. Although a transformational facilitator doesn't need formal credentials, he or she must be an expert in personal communications.

"I had been in traditional therapy for some time and had had a lot of success," explains Susan. "But I had gotten to a place where I wasn't moving forward, and I needed another way to look at myself. So I made an appointment to see Breck for some one-on-one work."

Breck worked out of a house in Santa Monica. "I remember showing up that day for an appointment," says Susan, "and expecting some wise old man to answer the door. So, when this combination Brad Pitt–Tom Cruise guy opened the door, the first thing I said was 'Okay, where's your dad?'"

One look at Breck and Susan was convinced it wasn't going to work. And nothing that occurred during the first session changed her mind.

"I found it difficult to understand what was going on," recalls Susan. "I thought, 'Yeah, maybe he'd be great to date, but that's it.'"

PUBLIC CONFESSION

In subsequent sessions, Breck introduced Susan to one of the underlying premises of transformational therapy—that we all have internal dialogues, or conversations, as Breck calls them, based on past experiences, that constantly run inside our heads. Revealing inner conversations takes the power away from these mental images.

"The way it was explained to me," says Susan, "is that when the conversation gets so loud that it demands your attention, it blocks you from hearing anything else. That's when it's time to 'go public' with it—revealing whatever the conversation is about.

"I knew part of the reason I was having difficulty understanding Breck was because [he] was [a] very attractive guy and I was a woman searching for a relationship. As a result, I began to role-play the way I thought a woman attracted to a man should be listening, rather than listening from a more authentic place."

The result was that Susan left the session not understanding anything Breck had said.

Back home, Susan reflected on her first hour with Breck. "I realized that the whole time I was there, all I was thinking was 'Gee, he's cute, I wonder if he's married?' and before I knew it I had this whole conversation going on inside my head that stopped me from hearing anything he had said."

Susan decided to go public—to reveal this inner conversation—at her next session with Breck. "I was really nervous but I confessed to him," Susan recalls. Susan also asked Breck if he was attracted to her. "He told me he was," Susan admits. But he also told her that the attraction was not the purpose of their relationship and that they should put aside those feelings and try to establish a deeper relationship.

Breck suggested that Susan might want to join a group of men and women who met with him three times a week from 7 to 9 A.M. "There would generally be about eight to twelve people, and we all sat around this big conference table," Susan recalls. "One by one we would get into discussions and Breck would work with us to help us understand the nature of our conversations."

Susan began to understand that some of her own internal conversations were related to the early days of her career. "When I broke on the scene in the seventies, everything was about being a sex symbol," explains Susan." It became a really strong part of my identity—dictating how I fit into the world, how I looked, and how I performed. I realized that it was really about trying to please everybody. I thought if I could just supply everybody with what they needed, then I would belong.

"But as I aged and evolved as a person I realized what *I* thought about me was more important than what other people thought. I was in conflict—part of me was living in the seventies and part [was living] in the nineties."

If Susan was going to have a breakthrough in her career, this conflicting internal image would have to break down. As Breck helped her separate what she was saying about her image and herself, things started to shift.

The result? "I grew up and stopped trying to figure out what everyone else wanted me to be and just started to run the risk of letting *me* emerge. Almost instantaneously, I got work and haven't been out of work for the past three and a half years. Even though I'm older and there's an overall recession, I'm making more money than ever," Susan says with glee.

But the long-term effect was even better. "I was again excited about my life and work," Susan says.

The effects were so uplifting that when the group she was in came to an end, she asked Breck if there was another one she could join. There was, of course, and Breck directed her to another group composed of actors, producers, and writers that met one evening per week.

Susan's intention was to focus on her work, but Breck encouraged her to work on her perception of male and female roles in society and its effect on her relationships.

While Susan was able to support herself financially, emotionally she was still looking for the man who could give her financial security and take care of her. "I was raised with the idea that the man is the provider and the woman is the nester," says Susan.

"I was still stuck in an old 'conversation,'" Susan admits. But her transformational work helped her to see it and wrench herself free.

"Breck showed me how to redirect where I was looking from, so that instead of looking for a guy to put a roof over my head, I was really looking for somebody with whom I could feel a sense of trust, honesty, and integrity," says Susan.

With this awareness, Susan was able to sift through the rubble from her conversations. As she did, she began to realize that Jeff Lester, a man who was also taking the seminar, was the man for whom she had been searching.

"He was standing there all along," recalls Susan, "but I couldn't see him at first because my vision was clouded by the fact that he didn't have a steady job or a big enough house. At that time, we were both struggling actors—just struggling at different levels."

Fortunately, "Breck helped me to see that Jeff was the man for me."

Although happily married today and with a career that's packing in audiences in Las Vegas, Susan admits that she is not totally free of the inner conversations.

But now she has the tools to deal with them. "Now when these conversations start," says Susan, "I recognize them for what they're worth and don't give them much weight. I could be watching television, for example, and a successful woman would start talking about her marriage and perfect life and all of a sudden I'd think, 'She has it all.' I'd covet that without realizing I was being shown just a fragment of her life. It would trigger an inner mechanism and all of a sudden I'd think my life isn't what I want. But then I'd realize that's not true.

"What I loved about this therapy," says Susan, "is that it comes from a place that says there's nothing wrong with any of us. We just need to rebalance our identity because it's our identity that dictates where we are going. If you are able to separate yourself from your identity, which is what you are helped to do, then you can really listen to yourself and get on course."

Today Susan is living her life full speed ahead with her eyes and ears wide open, making both professional and personal decisions from a very wise place.

It's been more than three years since Susan and Jeff married. After several highly successful years, they have settled in Las Vegas, Nevada, where Susan headlines at the Flamingo and Jeff successfully manages her ever-expanding career. Their commitment to transformational work continues. In fact, they have weekly phone consultations with Breck.

"Often we don't know what we are going to talk about," comments Susan. "But something always comes up. Transformational therapy is a lot like preventive medicine—it helps keep our eyes open and located on our inner truths."

SPOTLIGHT ON TRANSFORMATIONAL THERAPY

Imagine willfully agreeing to take a barefoot stroll over burning-hot coals or volunteering to stand up in front of 200 participants to act out the most negative aspects of your personality—all in an effort to improve your health, wealth, and overall well-being.

While engaging in these techniques and others like them may be beyond your comfort zone, thousands of people throughout the world sign up each day for these experiences in an effort to improve everything from their marriages, job, and bank accounts to their backs and blood pressure.

Frequently lumped together under the name "transformational therapy," the root of these experiences is the belief that the mind and the language we use to describe ourselves are powerful tools that can be programmed to help us reach maximum potential in all areas of life. Group facilitators—often thought of as human potential coaches—show us in both group and individual settings how the way in which we speak to ourselves and others can greatly affect our lives. Such seemingly benign phrases as "I'm *dying* for some time off," for example, are more likely to put us in a sickbed than on a sandy beach, sipping a fruity drink.

Transformational therapy traces its roots to humanistic psychology, a field of study that first came to public attention in the 1950s, when psychologist and educator Carl Rogers, Ph.D., began to conceptualize the human potential movement. Under this movement, techniques and training were created to take patients off the proverbial couch and onto more effective routes to attaining maximum physical and emotional health.

Sometime in the early- to mid-seventies, the human potential movement received its greatest forward push when personal growth seminars began to pop up, tackling a number of issues. Leading this parade was Werner Erhard's "EST Training," which had people flocking by the thousands to work with this highly motivational but controversial leader. Individuals were shown, through group and one-on-one procedures designed to break down the individual and rebuild a new self, how they could find *it*—it being an inner power that they viewed as the key to transforming their lives. They emerged from this transformational therapy claiming the ability to drop or lower their dependency on everything from mind-altering addictive substances to prescription eyeglasses, blood pressure medication, and even insulin.

These claims led professionals to question just how long the alleged results would last.

Today, the controversy remains, but you need take only one look at the best-seller lists and packed seminars across the country to discover how popular transformational therapy has become in recent years.

Whether it's Breck Costin's *Lifeworks Seminars*, *The Forum*, *Insight Transformational Seminars*, or even *Firewalking*, a personal growth experience that has participants walk over burning coals, the central element to all these transformational therapies is the role of the leader, who is often thought of as a consultant, coach, or facilitator.

While the methods each leader uses to enable participants to undergo a transformation vary—from teaching individuals the power of using healing words to engaging in wilderness training, where participants are pushed to physical limits in an effort to discover inner resources—all these leaders seem to possess some degree of charisma and a marked ability to inspire, motivate, and help individuals transform limiting beliefs into limitless possibilities. Participants often speak of the amount of personal freedom they experience by merely being in the presence of these human potential development coaches.

While many of these techniques need to be experienced through practitioners or in a group setting, one effective way to get started is by spending a day listening to the words you use. Researchers in these areas claim that the way in which we speak to ourselves and engage in conversations with others has a strong effect on our ability to do everything from heal to make money. Look at the way you use language. Are you literally *dying* to take a day off or constantly affirming that you *can't* get a job done, continually finding it on your to-do list, day after day? What about your tennis serve? Do you constantly remind yourself that you *just can't* get any better? Plan a mini vacation, start saying you *can* get it done, and tell yourself you have a solid tennis serve and see how that begins to affect your life.

Try this with behavior as well. The next time you find yourself *frozen in fear* about having to get up and talk before a group—fear that can cut off your creative juices and maybe even affect your immune system—try imagining that fear transforming into excitement. Work with your mind and senses. See the crowd smiling as you get on stage, reaching out to you with their approval and providing thunderous applause as you exit the stage. Now, that wasn't so bad, was it?

Keep in mind, however, that for depression and similar potentially dangerous illnesses, these programs are not a substitute for professional counseling. While many of these seminars are led by motivational leaders who may be certified in their particular therapy, they may be inexperienced in other areas, especially when it comes to your health. Any medical decisions about lowering your medications or changing a course of medical treatment should not be attempted without first consulting your primary health professional.

So if you're ready to experience a transformation, perhaps to gain greater personal endurance or to enhance your self-esteem, a good place to start is with extension courses offered through adult education programs at local universities, community centers, or the YMCA. Some may offer a free introductory class to give you a taste of what this alternative work is all about.

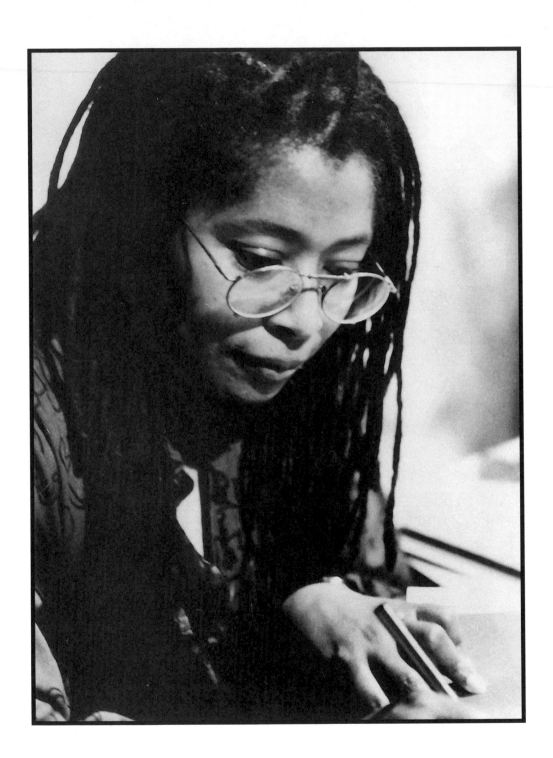

ALICE WALKER
AUTHOR

17 WATSU

BORN
1944, Eatonton, Georgia

EDUCATION
B.A., Sarah Lawrence College, 1965

PROFESSIONAL AWARDS
Pulitzer Prize, American Book Award, Townsend Prize, Lyndhurst Prize, Lillian Smith Award (National Endowment for the Arts), Rosenthal Award (National Institute of Arts and Letters), Radcliffe Institute Fellowship, Merrill Fellowship, Guggenheim Fellowship

CAREER HIGHLIGHTS
SELECTED NOVELS
The Color Purple
The Temple of My Familiar
Possessing the Secret of Joy
Warrior Marks

SELECTED POETRY
Goodnight
Willie Lee
I'll See You in the Morning
Horses Make a Landscape Look More Beautiful

CHILDREN'S BOOKS
Langston Hughes
To Hell with Dying

"The effects are forever when you have an encounter like this."

Fifty-year-old Alice Walker has published six novels, four volumes of poetry, two collections of short stories, two collections of essays, and two children's books. She won the Pulitzer Prize and the American Book Award for Fiction—both for her novel *The Color Purple*—and she produced the groundbreaking film *Warrior Marks*, a documentary on female genital mutilation.

One of the premier storytellers of our time, Alice Walker is equally renowned for her preference for privacy. So when Alice decides to talk, you can safely assume it is because she feels she has something important to contribute. It took just one watsu treatment for Alice to decide to share her personal experience.

It was Alice's great curiosity, openness and willingness to experiment that first led her to discover watsu, the water therapy that combines a soothing underwater massage with the free— and freeing—movement of water.

"I love to try new and interesting and possibly wonderful things," says Alice. "So I was intrigued by the idea of having a massage underwater—not really underwater, but in water up to my nose—with someone holding me and massaging me too."

Others who have tried watsu say it touches all dimensions of being—emotional, psychological, spiritual, and physical. They speak of reaching deep states of relaxation that allow them to let go at a level they've never before experienced. Some even say they feel as though they've floated all the way back to the womb and been reborn. Others let go of lifelong fears of water. Still others report energy surges and even spiritual awakenings. And many talk of releasing old traumas trapped within the body—freeing both heart and mind to love and trust once again.

How can a simple therapy have such wide-ranging effects? No one really knows. But watsu therapists feel that allowing yourself to float into a trance-like state with no one but a complete stranger to shelter and guide you builds a kind of trust and connectedness that seems to have far-reaching effects.

A NEW FORUM

Each person who experiences watsu works through emotions and feelings that are unique to their own experience. For Alice Walker, watsu became a new forum to grapple with the issues of bonding and trust—two themes that run throughout her work and life. No one, for example, could ever forget the trust that allowed Celie and her sister Nettie to stay connected in *The Color Purple*, and how every nuance of that feeling was explored and tested by time, distance, fathers, husbands, and bureaucrats.

But how did Alice come to further explore the complexity of trust through watsu?

"I was at a yoga retreat in northern California," explains Alice. "I was working on what I am always working on, which is trust. I was working on whether I could be in a new experience and be present in it and be fully there with the other person, but also be fully there with myself also."

Alice would be hard-pressed to think of a better way to expand her ability to trust. Or, for that matter, a better therapist to help her learn it. Because, fortunately for Alice, she was about to be massaged by the therapy's inventor, fifty-two-year-old massage therapist Harold Dull, a bushy-bearded graduate of San Francisco's poetry renaissance in the fifties.

After studying Zen shiatsu with master teachers in both the United States and Japan, Harold had returned to northern California to teach Zen shiatsu in 1980. While shiatsu involves the application of pressure through the hands and fingertips to various points on the body, Zen shiatsu builds on this to include various muscle stretches. Together, fingertip pressures and stretches are designed to increase flexibility, strengthen muscles, and unblock the channels through which *chi*—the Chinese term for personal energy or life force—flows.

But in California, Harold discovered that water amplifies the effects of shiatsu, both physically and emotionally. Moving the massage from land to water, he found he was now able to use the water's natural warmth and buoyancy to move the body into positions that would be impossible on land while, emotionally, the womblike water temperature created a feeling of safety, encouraging the person and their emotions to open up and flow.

The result? A feeling of complete trust between therapist and client.

SURRENDER YOUR FEELINGS

When Alice arrived at the retreat pool for her massage, she met Harold, who looks like a warm, well-hugged teddy bear. With a loving smile, the watsu therapist introduced himself to the author and began a poolside chat that would explain his therapy and begin to build a bond of trust.

"I was interested in the massage itself and not in the personality of the person who would be doing it," says Alice. "But I was happy that it was Harold Dull himself, since he had created this form of massage."

During their conversation, Alice was told that the basic principle behind watsu is to learn how to release emotions into the flow of surrounding water. She was told that it's common for a wide range of very deep emotions to surface during the therapy, and that by using the water and its natural movement, watsu is designed to give these stored or even locked-away feelings a way to emerge and be released from our bodies and souls. In most cases, Harold says, this will end their ability to keep us from fully experiencing life and robbing us of the natural power of life's energy.

Harold explained to Alice that if these emotions did start to surface, she should release them into the water's flow without trying to manage, examine, or rationalize them.

"The key word here is surrender," says Harold. "Whatever one is feeling should be surrendered into the flow."

Alice was told little more about what to expect because Harold wanted her to approach the experience without any preconceived notions. He did ask Alice about any expectations she had, however, and he asked whether she had any particular physical problems or fears of water. People who have circulation or heart problems, or even slipped disks, for example, may not be good candidates for therapy since the water in a watsu pool is warmed to 94°F. The heat can dilate arteries, increase circulation, and may tax an already challenged cardiovascular system. Or, it can aggravate swelling that is frequently associated with a slipped disk. If you have any medical problems at all, you should check with your doctor before trying any therapy that involves immersion in hot water.

Alice did possess a fear of getting into the water, but her fear was of Harold, not the water. "I'm not in the habit of getting into pools with strange men," Alice explains bluntly.

Once she had expressed her fear, however, Alice was free to move into the watsu massage. Having come that far, she was perfectly positioned to learn one of the lessons that watsu has to teach: to treat a specific emotion, even one as difficult as fear, simply as an awareness that can be released into the flow of life without any action. This is one of the most profound lessons that can be learned from watsu, Harold says.

Perhaps sensing this already, Alice followed Harold into the water. First he led her to the side of the pool and instructed her to touch the wall, telling her that this was the place where the session would both begin and end. Then he invited Alice into the deeper water.

For a few moments, he allowed Alice to simply stand in the pool, feeling the water's natural support. Then he began to demonstrate the Water Breath Dance, an exercise in which the client floats on the water's surface, allowing their breathing to move them higher and lower in the water. Harold uses the dance as a kind of punctuation throughout the watsu massage, allowing it to mark the end of each series of muscle stretches and massage that he completes. In that way, it also provides a much-needed sense of groundedness throughout what can be an otherwise disorienting experience.

"The Water Breath Dance shows how water lifts the body up as you breathe in and how you sink back into the water when you breathe out," explains Harold. "This is done with the head above water, feeling the role the water plays in lifting you in and out of it. It's an effortless surrender to water.

"I tell the client to close their eyes as I lift them to the surface," says Harold. "There they begin to float, feeling the natural rhythm of breath and the water. I put an arm under their tailbone and one of their arms behind my neck for additional support. Then I sink into the water and wait until I feel their body becoming lighter," an indication that they're relaxed.

It is here that the person being watsu'd and the therapist start to communicate simply through the rhythm of their bodies rather than through the spoken word.

"The Water Breath Dance moves me to a feeling state that connects me very deeply with the person I am working with," says Harold. "There is a stillness to the dance. And it is this stillness that is used to further establish trust between the therapist and the person who is receiving the massage." The stillness is so profound that the client enters into an altered state of consciousness, almost like a trance.

For the next hour Alice was floated and rocked in the warm water, supported by Harold's arms and body. There was no talk, only the rocking and swaying of their bodies as the massage progressed. Harold began with a gradual series of twists and turns that, if witnessed from a low-flying aircraft, might look like slow-moving underwater acrobatics. As Alice lay in his arms, Harold swung her knees open and closed, using one hand to support her head and keep it out of the water. Next he pulled her legs up toward her chest, then extended them back out along the water's surface once again. He rocked her hips from side to side.

Sometimes Harold would be standing behind Alice with her head lying back and resting on his shoulder; other times he would stand perpendicular to her floating body, supporting her head with his arms.

As watsu massage progresses, the body becomes more flexible and the movements become more complex and challenging. Eventually, the therapist is able to stand beside the person's floating body and stretch the legs over the head.

Between each of the different movements designed to increase flexibility, strengthen muscles, and release energy blocks in the body and emotional blocks in the spirit, there is a return, and a surrender, to the meditative stillness of the Water Breath Dance.

"It is the job of the massage therapist to hold the person being watsu'd, to support them, to float them into whatever they flow into," Harold says. "This profoundly affects people who have never experienced anyone being with them in this way—in an intimacy as deep as this without any need or intention attached to it. It allows them to experience what it feels like to have a oneness with someone they would never have imagined any connection with, teaching them that we are all truly one and connected.

"Once someone realizes that this connectedness is continual and does not depend on how well you know someone, the circumstances that brought you together, or how close you are physically, a powerful trust is established, reminiscent of that between a mother and child."

Harold suspects that the evolution of trust during watsu may be why the therapy seems to help victims of rape and incest. "Once someone is taught through watsu that it's okay to feel emotions and trust people, old hurts are released from the body," says Harold. "Yet all that is asked of each person being watsu'd is to give themselves as fully as they can to the experience—and to flow and relax into the arms of the person giving the massage."

THE PERSON WHO WALKS ON TWO FEET

It took a little more than an hour for Harold to complete Alice's watsu massage, but finally he led her back over to the side of the pool and placed her against it for support.

Once there against the wall, Alice knew it was her time to be alone and digest what she was feeling. "When the massage was finished, I was feeling very floaty," she says. "After all, here I was floating in this warm pool for an hour. I imagine that if the therapist had not been there to hold me and support me during that hour I would have just fallen to the bottom of the pool. So I took some time to collect myself and pull myself together—to be me again, the person who walks on two feet and is not floating in the water."

Harold adds: "Once I leave a person secured against the wall I make a clean separation. I stay in the water, in front of them, but without touching. And while we are no longer physically connected, the person still feels our inner connection. In fact, it's not uncommon for people who have undergone watsu to say that they continue to feel my support even though all physical contact has ceased. It is this feeling of support that is then carried out of the water by the client and into the world. It leaves the individual feeling that they are not alone—that they are still very deeply connected to a legacy of support. And many later tell me that this has been a very powerful and healing experience for them."

Alice might agree. She acknowledges the feeling of oneness and deep connection that the watsu massage encouraged. But watsu "also reconnected me with the kind of male energy that I had feared had almost disappeared from the earth," she adds. "From Harold, I felt the kind of male energy I knew from relatives as a child. The kind where, as a three-year-old, you were absolutely secure in the arms of strange men who would come in and lift you up and say, 'How are you?' and you would hug them and say, 'Fine.' You trusted them. To encounter a man and technique that has this type of affirming energy where it is not anything but supporting is incredible."

And just how long did these effects stay with Alice? "It's forever when you have an encounter like this where your trust is reaffirmed," Alice says.

"It's not as if you are discovering trust for the first time; it is something that is being reaffirmed, something you already know. You need to have it reaffirmed, you need to know that it still exists, that this particular wonderful thing you have found yet again is still around."

Or, as Harold Dull notes in his book *Watsu: Freeing the Body*, "...in water our bodies find the freedom the soul has lost."

SPOTLIGHT ON WATSU

Watsu is a massage therapy based on the ancient Japanese form of massage known as Zen shiatsu. It is conducted in a calm, waist-high pool of water warmed to a womblike 94°F.

In watsu, as in Zen shiatsu, a massage therapist stretches the limbs and applies pressure to various points along the body in an effort to release any tension that may be blocking the flow of *chi*, a kind of life force or energy. The result, its practitioners believe, is increased flexibility, stronger muscles, reduced stress, renewed energy, and even emotional healing.

Harold Dull, the inventor of watsu, studied shiatsu in Japan. Upon his return to the United States in 1980, he discovered that by moving the massage from land to water, he could increase the benefits offered by the massage. By using the warmth and natural buoyancy of water, for example, he could greatly increase the human body's flexibility and range of motion.

Harold called his new approach watsu because it described the technique's origins—"wat" for water and "su" for shiatsu. And although watsu is relatively new, Harold feels that it encourages the same benefits that have been ascribed to any form of hydrotherapy—increased circulation and relaxation, which can relieve pain and speed the healing of muscle and joint injuries and disabilities.

But watsu may have actually taken the healing principles of hydrotherapy one step further: Because watsu uses the Zen principle of continuous motion, a client receiving watsu cannot tense muscles in anticipation of a new move as an exercise begins and ends. This allows clients to reach deeper levels of mental and physical relaxation, Harold believes. It also gives the massage therapist the ability to take the client's body to a new level of flexibility.

As Harold's work began to evolve, it soon became evident that watsu also helps heal injured minds and spirits as well as injured bodies. The warm water, often described as womblike, provides a feeling of safety that allows recipients to release emotional blocks, including emotional traumas that have been locked inside for years.

Using the warm water as a natural cradle and supported by the arms and body of the massage therapist, the client is massaged and led through a series of stretches as he or she is rocked and floated in a pool for approximately an hour. It is up to the therapist to hold the person's head safely out of water.

There is great emphasis placed on breathing during the massage as the massage therapist works in harmony with the client's natural breathing rhythms to move the client into deeper levels of relaxation. With each stretch of the body, a breath is taken to complement the move. In a movement called the accordion, for example, the client's legs and head are brought together as the client breathes out, then extended back out across the water's surface as the client breathes in.

Ready to try watsu for yourself? Fortunately, the basics of watsu can be learned in as little as a weekend by almost anyone. With the help of a video and instruction manual prepared by Harold Dull, anyone lucky enough to have a heated pool and a cooperative partner can experience these massages without having to travel to an expensive spa.

Watsu advocates stress that it is truly as much fun to give watsu as it is to receive it, so before long this hard-to-find massage may be as close to home as your neighbor's pool.

If you have any preexisting medical problems, be sure to check with your doctor before entering any pool that's heated to 94°F, as is a watsu pool.

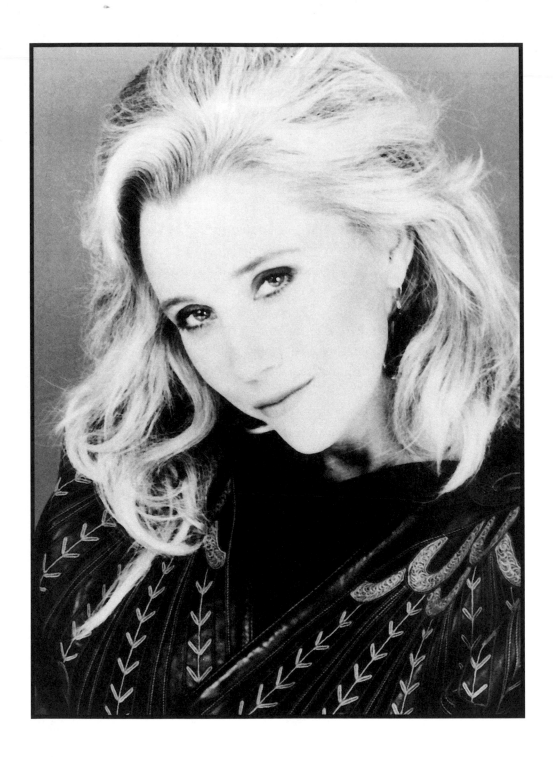

18 YOGA

BORN
October 31, 1944, New York, New York

EDUCATION
Lee Strasberg Theater Institute in Los Angeles; Integra Yoga Institute; The Actor's Studio

PROFESSIONAL AWARDS
Golden Globe nomination, Best Actress, 1992; Academy Award nomination, Best Actress, 1988; Golden Globe, Best Actress, 1988: *Anna*; Independent Spirit Award, Best Actress, 1988; Los Angeles Film Critics Award, Best Actress, 1988.

CAREER HIGHLIGHTS
SELECTED FILMS
JFK
Anna
Private Benjamin
A Star Is Born
The Way We Were
The Sting

SELECTED THEATER
Largo Desolato
Tom Paine, Where Has Tommy Flowers Gone?
Sweet Eros
Step on a Crack

"If I had not found yoga, I can truthfully say that I would be dead today. Yoga led me from a painful path of self-destruction onto a joyful path of self-exploration and, ultimately, self-enlightenment."

Today Sally Kirkland is a vibrant, energetic woman who has earned the highest honors an actor can. She's been nominated for an Academy Award for Best Actress, and as a result of her compelling portrait of a Czechoslovakian expatriate in the film *Anna*, she won the Golden Globe award for Best Actress in a Motion Picture.

But just about twenty-five years ago, Sally Kirkland lay unconscious in the emergency room of a New York City hospital, the victim of a massive, deliberate drug overdose that she hoped would end her life.

"It's a miracle that I'm alive today," says Sally. "When someone takes more than forty codeine tablets and sixty-five Nembutals like I did, they normally don't survive. Those are major, *major* tranquilizers. The doctors told my mother and father, 'Pray that she doesn't make it because she'll be a vegetable.'"

Fortunately, the on-duty physician refused to give up on the vulnerable young woman who lay in front of him. Pulling out all the stops, this doctor gave Sally another chance at life.

"QUEEN OF THE UNDERGROUND"

How a talented woman like Sally Kirkland fell into suicidal despair—and how she eventually turned her life around—reads like the script for one of those dramatic, emotional movies in which Sally acts up a storm.

At first glance, she certainly didn't seem a likely candidate for suicide. She was raised on Manhattan's wealthy Upper East Side by a father who hailed from Philadelphia's patrician Main Line and a mother, also named Sally Kirkland, who was a major player in the fashion scene of the forties, fifties, and sixties as fashion editor of *Vogue* and *Life*.

Often, the trendsetters of the moment could be found lounging around the spacious Kirkland apartment on the corner of 89th Street and Madison Avenue, just around the corner from the Guggenheim Museum of Art. "I'd come home from school and there in my living room would be the top super-models of the sixties like Verushka and Jean Shrimpton, laughing it up with designers like Bill Blass and Giorgio d'SantAngelo," says Sally.

It was a stimulating environment even though her parents were alcoholic. But eventually, Sally grew tired of that sophisticated, uptown world and headed for the artsy, downtown scene in Greenwich Village.

"I wanted to be a star, an artist, the next Marilyn Monroe," explains Sally. So "I went from living in a fabulous doorman building to a tiny walkup apartment with the bathtub in the kitchen."

Her timing was perfect. The cultural revolution known as "the sixties" was just about to explode, and Sally Kirkland would soon become "Queen of the Underground"—an outspoken, rebellious star in the brand-new world of Off-Broadway theater and art films.

Sally hurled herself headfirst into a new world of ego, glamour, and illusion. She shed her clothes on the New York City stage in the play *Sweet Eros* and, in an instant, went from studying Shakespearean acting with legendary teacher Joseph Papp to emoting in public without even a couplet of covering.

The controversy was stunning: She was the theater's first nude actor. But, "to me nudity was a political thing," says Sally. "I was making a statement against violence, war, and Vietnam." As Sally said at the time: "You can't carry a gun on a naked body."

The next thing she knew, Sally was one of Andy Warhol's first protegees, starring in his early underground movie, *The Thirteen Most Beautiful Women in the World.*

But there was a dark side to all this success, and Sally succumbed to it. "I started to drink too much, smoke too much," says Sally. "I took too many uppers and downers." She also began experimenting with the mind-altering drug LSD. In fact, Sally had the dubious distinction of being among the first wave of her generation to start "tripping." Unfortunately, a series of "bad trips" left Sally fixated on death. All streams of light, hope, and joy disappeared from her life, sucked into a "black hole" of dark, daily hallucinations. In particular, she became obsessed with Marilyn Monroe, especially the star's emotional pain and her suicide. Sally began to wear an actual pair of Marilyn's shoes everywhere she went. The shoes had been a gift to Sally from her friend Shelley Winters, who had once been Marilyn's roommate. Along with the shoes, Sally took on Monroe's mantle of despair and depression. And the more acid she consumed, the more her psyche was consumed by thoughts of self-destruction. Eventually Sally decided that she was destined not just to wear Marilyn's shoes but to follow in her footsteps and snuff out her own life.

"I remember going to my parents' apartment," says Sally. "I went into the bathroom and swallowed my mother's entire summer's supply of sleeping pills and painkillers. That's how I ended up in the emergency room."

FIFTEEN MINUTES IN PHILADELPHIA

Having survived a suicide attempt, Sally stayed in first one, then another of Manhattan's hospitals for treatment of her emotional health. But she didn't agree with the treatment offered by physicians there. "The doctors tried to convince me that I should never act again. They told me that I was too sensitive to handle the profession."

Sally wasn't about to abandon her life in the theater, no matter what the doctors said. Besides, she flat-out didn't buy their diagnosis. To Sally, it was her drug abuse, not her sensitivity, that had caused her to turn those glamorous Marilyn Monroe fantasies into a self-destructive reality. And if she could just get herself away from the outrageous lifestyle of the 'rebel star,' perhaps she could get away from drugs. Then, Sally was convinced, she might have a shot at a sane life.

Fortunately, events conspired to help her, and a theater company in Philadelphia asked Sally to join them.

"The first day at the Philadelphia theater the director told us, 'There's one thing you need to know. I don't want anyone to be in this theater company unless you understand that everyone of us is going to do yoga together every day.'"

That day, Sally took her first yoga class.

"I don't know how to describe what I felt except to say it was like I had an orgasm—except with my entire body, my entire being."

At the time, Sally was smoking two packs of cigarettes a day as she tried to kick the booze and drugs. "Suddenly I was doing this yoga exercise called the Breath of Fire, where you forcefully exhale air through your nose. We did maybe eighty or a hundred exhalations to start the class. I could literally taste the nicotine coming out of my lungs.

"When we finished all those exhalations, the teacher told us to inhale and hold our breath. She said that the toxins in our body were being burned up, and that when we finally exhaled, a lot of that toxicity would be removed. I remember, she said, 'You'll have a lot of energy.'

"Well, that was an understatement! I never felt anything like it! My whole body was buzzing with life."

Sally's joy only increased as the class progressed.

"By the time we were doing the deep relaxation exercises at the end of the class, I was in heaven! I felt like my whole body was smiling.

"The teacher told us to lie completely still and not move our bodies, no matter what. At first, I wanted to scratch myself or move around, because I wasn't used to just being quiet and still. But the teacher said that if we remained still, we would learn that our bodies do not run us. Instead, we would find that our minds are really in control of our bodies. And, likewise that we could learn to still our minds. I remember thinking about the line from the Bible, 'Peace, be still.'

"The deep relaxation exercise at the end of a yoga class usually lasts about fifteen minutes. Well, during those fifteen minutes in Philadelphia I was quiet and still for the first time in my life, without having to be asleep!

"One of my most desperate prayers for help had been answered. Finally, I was experiencing peace of mind.

"If someone had said to me at the moment I was lying there, 'You're an actor, right? And you want to be a movie star?' I would have said, 'Forget it, I'm into this.'"

THE HEALING GIFT

No longer driven by her quest for fame, Sally felt a tremendous sense of release.

As she did her daily yoga exercises with the Philadelphia theater company, she became calmer and more relaxed. Her desire for cigarettes, alcohol, and drugs melted away, and she decided to dedicate herself to learning as much as she could about yoga. If yoga could free her from the yoke of addictions, she thought, what other benefits could there be?

For the next two years, Sally immersed herself in the world of yoga. She was first a student, then a student and teacher at the internationally acclaimed Integral Yoga Institute in New York.

The physical benefits were astounding.

"My whole body became flexible really fast. I was able to bend forward, put my head on my knees, chest on my thighs, and my hands at my feet. Now that's a tough one."

Increased flexibility is one of the wonderful benefits that all of us can get from yoga, no matter what our level of fitness or age, says Sally.

"I had one man in my yoga class who was ninety-five years young! He was incredible, doing headstands and everything."

Sally doesn't hesitate to tell anyone and everyone of the physical benefits she's reaped from the practice of yoga. But that's not all she's gained from this alternative method of achieving balanced health. One of the greatest gifts of yoga, she says, is how it helped her become more open to the spiritual dimension of everyday life.

In fact, Sally believes that the inner peace she's found through yoga may be the most profoundly healing gift she received from this ancient science. Like many people who are avid practitioners, Sally says that her ability to find a sense of peace inside herself is the greatest tool she's gotten from yoga. Why? It's the key she uses to handle the daily stress that might otherwise make drugs and booze look appealing.

How did Sally find this inner peace, this spiritual source so powerful that she credits it with saving her life?

She pauses for a long, reflective moment before answering the question. When she does speak, her voice is filled with contentment and serenity.

"The bottom line of yoga is the understanding that 'We are all one,'" she says. "You know, the word *yoga* means 'union.' That means that there is no separation between you or me in the spiritual sense. My soul and your soul are, in truth, one. We may have different personalities or different karma to work out, but the common denominator between us is the truth that we are one. A profound healing love comes from your awareness of that truth."

How can the rest of us tap into this power of universal love?

"To achieve spiritual awareness through yoga," she says, "the first thing you want to do is to let go of anything that separates you from anyone else—whether it's race, creed, color, religion, whatever. Yoga has to do with loving *all* of God's creation. This is a big part of the philosophy of yoga—we cannot judge each other because everything that exists in *me* exists in *you*.

"I believe that we all have God inside us. We have a higher consciousness, if you will. That doesn't mean that everybody has to believe in God. It just means that everyone has to start recognizing that we all have joy and we all suffer."

This spiritual belief in "individual peace" generated through yoga is a cornerstone of Sally's resurrected life. She swears its limitless power brought her back to life, restored her to sanity, and continues to keep her alive today.

Twenty-five years after her first yoga class, Sally says she continues to practice and teach yoga with a zeal approaching devotion. And today Sally's own personal energy seems boundless. Besides acting, she directs, produces, paints, composes poetry, lectures on spiritual inner awareness, and teaches the Sally Kirkland Acting Workshops all over the world.

"The two things I hear most in my life are Where do you get your energy from? and How come you look so young? And I have to honestly say that it's from yoga. Because I have been doing yoga since 1969, and in many ways I feel a whole lot younger than when I started."

SPOTLIGHT ON YOGA

What do famous names Raquel Welch, Kareem Abdul-Jabbar, and Sting have in common? Yoga!

"I want to reduce the amount of stress in my life. I've seen it kill my parents. I've seen it kill friends. I don't want it."

Believe it or not, that's Sting talking, the man who used to write rock classics like "King of Pain" by living the part.

But not anymore. "I used to believe that you had to be destructive to be creative. I don't want to do that anymore, I want to lead a quiet, well-adjusted life and still be creative."

Part of his plan is yoga, which Sting uses to attain inner peace as well as his famous taut and well-toned body. He practices the ancient art in his dressing room every night before taking the stage. In fact, at a concert in Paris a few years ago, he was spotted backstage sitting in a full lotus position—wearing only the tiniest of bikini briefs and a court jester's hat. (Guess you can't take *all* the rock and roll out of the master, no matter how hard he tries!)

Raquel Welch, whose physique most women would love to have, includes yoga as part of her regular fitness program, and appears on videotape in yoga workouts designed to keep the shapely parts shapely and the tight parts tight.

Kareem Abdul-Jabbar, the basketball legend, is an athlete almost unmatched in strength, skill, and focus. Like many athletes, Kareem uses yoga to help stay limber, recover from injuries, and stay focused.

Yoga is a series of physical positions, breathing exercises, and focused concentration that is designed to unite body, mind, and spirit into an integrated whole. One of the side effects of this unity is a healing peace that neutralizes the health-damaging effects of the physical and mental stress caused by injury, disease, and emotional turmoil. That's why today, yoga is a small but important part of treatment for everything from arthritis to AIDS.

One physician who prescribes yoga is Andrew Weil, M.D., a graduate of Harvard Medical School and author of *Natural Health, Natural Medicine*. Dr. Weil is a practicing physician in Tucson, Arizona, who is an adviser to a government study on alternative cancer therapies. What's his opinion of yoga?

"Yoga is an excellent way to strengthen the back, balance nervous functioning, promote flexibility, and neutralize stress," reports Dr. Weil.

Another physician who prescribes yoga is medical pioneer Dean Ornish, M.D., author of the best-selling *Reversing Heart Disease*. Dr. Ornish has actually used yoga as part of a heart-healthy program that includes a strict vegetarian diet, daily exercise, no smoking, and lots of hugs. His approach has been known to reverse many of the risk factors—high cholesterol and high blood pressure, for example—that are known to damage arteries and cause heart attacks.

Yoga evolved in India out of a religious tradition around the second century B.C. It developed among a group of people who had devoted their lives to the attainment of spiritual insight. The yogis—as these spiritual leaders came to be called—developed a method that would unite the physical, emotional, and intellectual elements of each person. The word *yoga* means "join together" or "unite" in Sanskrit, the yogis' native language.

There are different styles of yoga, but if you're looking for health benefits, check out "hatha yoga." This is the style of yoga that emphasizes relaxation through breathing and stretching. The purpose of hatha yoga is to completely relax, giving you control over your mind. While you're in this relaxed state, you can tone your body and soothe your emotions.

Yoga exercises are done on a flat surface with plenty of space to stretch your arms and legs in all directions. It's best to use a large towel, mat, or pad under your body for comfort. Yoga is not a hurried affair. As a matter of fact, it almost appears that people doing yoga are moving in slow motion. As yoga expert Richard Hittleman says, "Yoga exercises are performed in a series of graceful, rhythmic movements—with a brief 'holding' period that's completely motionless for certain positions. Poise and balance are maintained at all times and the attention is fixed unwaveringly on the movements being executed.

"We attempt to approach each session in a serene frame of mind, having put aside all thoughts and activities that might be distracting," he says.

A great way to get acquainted with yoga is to enroll in a class. Many health clubs and YMCAs now offer classes. But until you discover a class for yourself, here are some quick tips that will introduce you to yoga's stress-relieving benefits:

If you find yourself tensing up in your car during a traffic jam, place one finger alongside your nose and close off one nostril. Take a deep, slow breath in and out through the other nostril. Switch nostrils and repeat. (Remember, you're still in traffic, so keep your eyes open.)

Feeling fatigued while you're in the kitchen cooking dinner? Spread your feet shoulder-width apart. Then take whatever kitchen utensils you're using—say, a spatula in one hand and the lid of a pot in the other—and slowly stretch your arms above your head, one at a time. Remember to breathe in deeply as you raise your arms, and out as you bring them back to your side.

Finally gotten to bed after a hectic day? While lying on your back, place your hands behind your head, with your elbows bent. Bend your knees, keeping your feet flat on the mattress. Slowly drop both knees to one side, breathing in and out deeply through your nostrils. Bring your knees back up straight, then drop them to the other side, continuing the deep breathing.

ACKNOWLEDGMENTS

Authors, like other humans, seem to function best when surrounded with love and support. During the writing of this book, I had the great fortune to be gifted with an almost embarrassingly large supply of both. For this I wish to acknowledge:

My spirited team of cheerleaders, Agapi Stassinopoulos, Alexandra McMullen, and Rama Fox. I can't say enough about the healing power of friendship.

Arielle Ford for her wisdom, compassion, and remarkable Rolodex.

Dr. Marc Rosenbaum, whose willingness to lend a caring and compassionate ear never ceases to amaze me.

Drs. Ron and Mary Hulnick for their wisdom in creating a University dedicated to the healing power of love and their courage in taking me on as a graduate student. They truly made school everything I always wished it could be and more.

Allan Hirsh III, Laura Wallace, Kathy Cash, and all those behind-the-scenes folks at Ottenheimer for their valuable contributions.

My editor Deborah Thornton Pendleton for her patience and guidance and Claire Gerus for her vision.

David Epstein, Steve Small, Geoffrey Menen, Chuck Baier, and Genie Ford for always showing up at the right time to provide a helping hand.

The Office of Alternative Healing for their heartfelt efforts to make alternative healing available to us all.

My research assistants Mitchell Brozinsky and Melanie Roth for their incredibly helpful attitudes and countless trips here and there for just one more bit of information.

Dr. Ed Wagner for his willingness to be available way beyond sane office hours.

Essum Khashoggi, Simon Hodgson, and the staff at EKI for keeping Laird so busy he never got to notice just how obsessed I became in getting this book done.

Nicholas Brown for a sanctuary to write this book in.

My beloved teacher and friend John-Roger, who has taught me more than any other person about the power of prayer and how sweet life can be.

To John Morton for his vision and rock-solid integrity.

To my nephews Joseph and Michael, for their useful energy.

To my father Harold Mintzer, for his deep wisdom, and my mother, Ethel, for passing on her willingness to always try something new.

To all of the dedicated secretaries, assistants, public relations staff, and agents I worked with to bring this book together.

And finally to the eighteen celebrated people whose stories of healing and courage I had the privilege to listen to—for their willingness to share what worked for them in the hope that it might inspire someone else to create a happier and healthier life.

WHERE TO FIND OUT MORE

Author's note: Whenever possible, seek out the recommendation of one or more people when using any alternative health practitioner.

ACUPUNCTURE

Make sure that any acupuncturist you use has a minimum of two years' training at an accredited acupuncture school. Your local schools of Chinese and Oriental medicine will generally provide a list of graduates to choose from.

Some states, but not all, require acupuncturists to be certified by the National Commission for the Certification of Acupuncturists. A list of those who are certified can be obtained by calling the NCCA at (202) 232-1404 in Washington, D.C.

You may wish to turn to one of the 3,000 or so M.D.s in the United States who are both acupuncturists and medical doctors. To find one near you, call the American Academy of Medical Acupuncture at (800) 521-2262.

AYURVEDIC MEDICINE

If you're interested in consulting with an ayurvedic physician, contact the Center for Mind/Body Medicine in La Hoya, California, at (619) 794-2425.

CHINESE HERBAL MEDICINE

To find a Chinese herbal medicine practitioner near you, call the American Foundation of Traditional Chinese Medicine at (202) 966-7338, or in

California, call The Center for Regeneration at (310) 271-6467. The American Botanical Council in Austin, Texas, (800) 373-7105, may be able to help you find information on any herbs that may be prescribed.

COLON HYDROTHERAPY

To find a colon hydrotherapist in your area, contact the International Association for Colon Hydrotherapy at (916) 222-1497.

CREATIVE VISUALIZATION

The Academy for Guided Imagery in Mill Valley, California, (415) 389-9324, can refer you to practitioners in your area who use creative visualization in their practice.

ENVIRONMENTAL MEDICINE

Many alternative practitioners—doctors of Oriental medicine, acupuncturists, chiropractors—have a subspecialty in environmental medicine, so check with your practitioner for further advice in this area.

FENG SHUI

Read a book or take a class at your local college or community center, or contact the Lin Yun Temple in Berkeley, California, (510) 841-2347.

HOMEOPATHY

To find a homeopath near you, call the National Center for Homeopathy in Alexandria, Virginia, at (703) 548-7790. Other organizations that may provide information or referrals include the International Foundation for Homeopathy in Seattle, Washington, at (206) 324-8230, and the American Institute of Homeopathy in Denver, Colorado, at (303) 898-5477. Since many people practice homeopathic medicine with no formal degrees, there are kits available through: Homeopathic Educational Services, 2124 Kittredge Street, Berkeley, California 94704; (415) 649-0294.

JUICING

If you have difficulty locating books or juicing machines at your local health food store, you may want to call Get Juiced at (800) 537-7010, a company in New York City that will express-deliver prepared juices to you in time for breakfast.

MACROBIOTICS

For more information about macrobiotics, contact the Kushi Institute, a non-profit organization founded by Michio Kushi in Becket, Massachusetts, (413) 623-5741.

MASSAGE

If you're curious about the latest developments in this ever-expanding field, your local newsstand might just have a copy of *Massage Therapy Journal* or *Massage Magazine*. Or call the American Massage Therapy Association in

Evanston, Illinois, at (312) 761-2682. To contact a Rubenfeld Surgerist in your area, contact the Rubenfeld Center in New York City, (212) 254-5100.

MIND/BODY MEDICINE

To find out how you can incorporate these techniques as part of a preventive health-care program or as an adjunct treatment to more conventional medical care, contact the Center for Mind/Body Studies in Washington, D.C., at (202) 966-7338, or the Mind/Body Medical Institute in Boston, directed by Herbert Benson, M.D., a key researcher in mind/body medicine, at (617) 632-9525.

ROLFING

To find a Rolfer in your area, contact the Rolf Institute at (800) 530-8875, Boulder, Colorado.

TRANSFORMATIONAL THERAPY

Contact the University of Santa Monica for a complete program of workshops at (310) 829-7402. Breck Costin's Lifeworks Seminars are based in Los Angeles, California. Call (213) 655-6008 for specific trainings in your area. Insight Educational Seminars are presented throughout the world; contact (800) 656-9385.

WATSU

In the United States, Watsu is available at the Two Bunch Palms spa located near Palm Springs, California; the Ten Thousand Waves spa in Santa Fe,

New Mexico; and at Harbin Hot Springs in northern California, where Harold Dull first developed the technique. But, given its fast-growing popularity, you may check with your local health spa, or call Harbin Hot Springs at (707) 987-2477 for additional locations.

YOGA

If you're interested in a formal yoga program but can't seem to find one, call the *Yoga Journal* at (510) 841-9200. They can hook you up with a class in your area. Or call the Himalayan Institute of Yoga, Science and Philosophy in Honesdale, Pennsylvania, at (800) 822-4547. The institute sponsors classes at centers all over the country. And for further information on yoga as a therapy, contact the International Association of Yoga Therapists in Mill Valley, California, at (415) 383-4587. A nonprofit organization devoted to yoga education and research, the association produces the *Journal of the International Association of Yoga Therapists.*

RECOMMENDED READING LIST

ACUPUNCTURE

Plain Talk About Acupuncture, Ellinor R. Mitchell, published by Whalehall.

AYURVEDIC MEDICINE

Perfect Health: The Complete Mind Body Guide, Deepak Chopra, M.D., published by Harmony Books.
Quantum Healing, Deepak Chopra, M.D., published by Bantam Books.

BEE POLLEN THERAPY

Royden Brown's Bee Hive Product Bible, Royden Brown, published by Avery Publishing Group.

CHINESE HERBAL MEDICINE

Between Heaven and Earth: A Guide to Chinese Medicine, Harriet Beinfeld, published by Ballantine Books.

COLON HYDROTHERAPY

The Hippocrates Health Program, Brian R. Clement, published by Hippocrates Publications.
Colon Health: Key to a Vibrant Life, Norman Prescott Walker, published by Norwalk Press.

CREATIVE VISUALIZATION

Creative Visualization, Shakti Gawain, published by New World Library.
Staying Well with Guided Imagery: How to Harness the Power of Your Imagination for Health and Healing, Belleruth Naparstek, published by Warner Books.
The Power Within You, John Roger, published by Mandeville Press.

ENVIRONMENTAL MEDICINE

No More Allergies: Identifying and Eliminating Allergies and Sensitivity Reactions to Everything in Your Environment, Gary Null, published by Villard Books.

FENG SHUI

Interior Design with Feng Shui, Sarah Rossbach, published by Penguin Books.
The Feng Shui Handbook: A Practical Guide to Chinese Geomancy and Environmental Harmony, Derek Walters, published by The Aquarian Press.

HOMEOPATHY

Homeopathic Medicine at Home: Natural Remedies for Everyday Ailments & Minor Injuries, Maesimund Panos and Jane Heimlich, published by G.P. Putnam and Sons.

JUICING

Juicing for Life: A Guide to the Health and Benefits of Fresh Juice and Vegetable Juicing, Cherie Calbom & Maureen Keane, published by Avery Publishing Group.

MACROBIOTICS

Adventures of a Kamikaze Cowboy, Dirk Benedict, published by Avery Publishing Group.
Macrobiotic Diet, Michio & Aveline Kushi, published by Japan Publications.
A Guide to Healthy Cuisine: Mostly Macro for the Discriminating Palate, Lisa Turner, published by Healing Arts Press.

MASSAGE

The Book Of Massage, Lucinda Lidell, published by Fireside Publishers.
Therapeutic Touch, Dorothy Krieger, published by Bear & Company.

MIND/BODY MEDICINE

Body, Mind & Spirit: A Guide to Fitness, John Douillard, published by Harmony Books.

Minding the Body, Mending the Soul, Joan Borysenko, published by Warner Books.

Reversing Heart Disease, Dean Ornish, M.D., published by Ballantine Books.

The Art of Breathing: A Course of Six Simple Lessons to Improve Performance and Well Being, Nancy Zi, published by Vivi Company.

MEDITATION

Inner Worlds of Meditation, John Roger, published by Mandeville Press.

PSYCHIC SURGERY

Healers & The Healing Process: A Report on 10 Psychic Surgeons, George W. Meek, published by Quest Books.

Healing Words: The Power of Prayer Therapy, Larry Dossey, M.D., published by Harper San Francisco.

ROLFING

The Integration of Human Structure, Ida Rolf, published by Harper & Row.

TRANSFORMATIONAL THERAPY

Unlimited Power, Anthony Robbins, published by Ballantine Books.

WATSU

Freeing the Body in Water, Harold Dull, published by Harbin Springs
  Publishing.

YOGA

Yoga For Health, Richard Hittleman, published by Ballantine Books.
Power Yoga: The Total Strength and Flexibility Workout, Beryl Bender Birch,
  published by Fireside Publishers.